CARDIAC TRANSPLANTATION

Edited by **Susan D. Moffatt-Bruce**

Cardiac Transplantation
Edited by Susan D. Moffatt-Bruce

Published by InTech
Janeza Trdine 9, 51000 Rijeka, Croatia

Publishing Process Manager Marija Radja

Technical Editor Teodora Smiljanic

Cover Designer InTech Design Team

Additional hard copies can be obtained from orders@intechopen.com

Cardiac Transplantation, Edited by Susan D. Moffatt-Bruce
p. cm.
ISBN 978-953-51-0000-3

For EU product safety concerns:
IN TECH d.o.o., Prolaz Marije Krucifikse Kozulić 3, 51000 Rijeka, Croatia,
info@intechopen.com or visit our website at intechopen.com.

Meet the editor

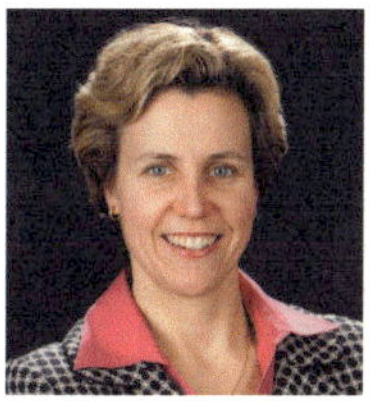

Dr Susan Moffatt-Bruce is a board certified cardiothoracic surgeon and the Chief Quality and Patient Safety Officer at the Ohio State University Medical Center. She completed her undergraduate degree at McGill University. Having successfully completed Dalhousie Medical School Dr Moffatt-Bruce competed for and was awarded a residency position in General Surgery at Dalhousie University. She secured the Killam Postgraduate Research Award, the Overseas Research Student Award (University of Cambridge) and the Cambridge Commonwealth Trust Bursary Award. She was the first surgical resident at Dalhousie University to complete her Ph.D. during residency training. She was awarded the Bayer-Canadian Association of Allergy and Clinical Immunology Research Award, the British Transplantation Society Research Award and the Sackler Scholarship. She was the Cardiothoracic Surgery fellow at Stanford University and was on staff at the University of British Columbia, before being recruited to OSUMC. She has become NIH funded with an active laboratory in transplantation research and also developed a passion for Quality and Patient Safety initiatives and process improvement. Dr Moffatt-Bruce lives in Columbus, Ohio with her husband Nigel and their two girls, Emily and Sarah.

Contents

Preface

The completion of this book is very exciting as we consider all the innovations around cardiovascular healthcare world wide. We are truly in an era of change not only in terms of technology but in the type of patient we are caring for. With change come challenges around truly multidisciplinary management of transplant patients. That is why I feel this book is exciting in that it presents the team approach to the transplant patient. I am confident that the pioneers of cardiac transplantation would be pleased with our response to challenges in healthcare today and be pleased with the final product. I would like to thank Dr. Bruce Reitz, my neverending supporter and mentor who started me on this journey.

Susan D. Moffatt-Bruce, MD, PhD
Chief Quality and Patient Safety Officer,
Associate Professor of Surgery,
Ohio State University Medical Center,
USA

Part 1

Treatment Strategies in Cardiac Transplantation

1

Immunosuppressive Therapy After Cardiac Transplantation

Martin Schweiger
Medical University Graz, Department for Surgery,
Division for Transplantation Surgery,
Austria

1. Introduction

In contrast to renal or pancreas transplantation graft failure after heart transplantation (HTx) is associated with the death of the patient if re-grafting or mechanical support (MCS) is not possible immediately. Since the beginning of modern transplantation medicine one of the highest priorities were preventing and treating graft rejection. Over the last decades experimental, animal and clinical research resulted in the development of new immunosuppressive (IS) drugs leading to an improved patient and graft survival. The efforts of transplant professions to develop new IS protocols trying to reduce the toxic side effects, resulted in an improvement of quality of life (QoL) for transplant recipients.

2. Historical consideration

At the beginning of the twentieth century research work by Alexis Carrel on performing surgical anastomosis [1, 2] allowed organ revascularization and marked one of the pre-conditions for organ transplantation. It was the Stanford group of Lower and Shumway who first started to study the problems of HTx [3-5] leading to the first human HTx by Banard in 1967 [6]. Within the next year over 100 HTx were done worldwide. Even if technical successful the great enthusiasm for this new therapy decreased rapidly when the poor survival rate became obvious [7]. One of the biggest problem was preventing and controlling graft rejection. Corticosteroides and Azathioprine (AzA) were the main drugs used for IS at that time. The Standford group added rabbit antithymocyte globulin (ATG) to the protocol gaining acceptable survival rates [8]. The main breakthrough came a decade later with a drug called Cyclosporine (CsA). The great advantage of CsA was the selective immunoregulation of T cells in contrast to the non-selective inhibition of cell proliferation by AzA and corticosteroids. CsA was first used in clinical organ transplantation in 1978 [9] and in 1983 it was approved for clinical use to prevent graft rejection in transplantation. Today transplant professions throughout the world contribute the great success of HTx to the introduction of CsA into clinical practice. Four years after the first use of CsA Kino reported of a new IS agent even more potent compared to CsA called FK 506 [10]. It was Starzl and the Pittsburgh Group who but much effort in the establishment of FK 506 into IS protocols [11]. In the recent FK 506 is more frequently used compared to CsA [12].

As early as 1896, mycophenolate acid (MPA), the activated form of mycophenolate mofetil (MMF) was extracted from Penicillium stoloniferum (Gosio, B. 1896. Ricerche batteriologiche chimiche sulle alterazioni del mais. Riv. Igiene Sanita Pub. Ann.7:825-869. 16. Jaureguiberry). The cytostatic effect was reported by Brewin in 1972 and was first used in the treatment of neoplasia [13]. The first report of MMF use as IS drug in animal research was in a heterotopic HTx model in rats [14].

Lately a new category named proliferation signal inhibitors (PSI), including Rapamycin (Rapa) and Everolimus (EvE) have been introduced to clinical practice. Rapa was discovered in 1965 but it took years before it was introduced to transplantation medicine. The research work of Rapa led to the discovery of the action of the mammalian target of Rapamycin (mTOR).

3. Immunosuppressive regimes and agents

Starting with the exploration of CsA the field of IS agents has evolved drastically resulting in the possibility of more combinations for different indications. All IS agents have a narrow therapeutic window in common. Transplant physicians have to find an optimal balance avoiding allograft rejection and avoid toxic side effects. There are mainly three categories for IS therapy: first its use as induction therapy, second to maintain the organ allograft (maintenance therapy) and finally if needed to treat acute rejection episodes (anti-rejection therapy). In the following we focus on the recent used IS agents, acting at T cell mediated processes of rejection. Further agents focusing on the role of antibody mediated rejection may be found in the next chapter.

The highest number of rejection episodes will be within the first months after HTx; therefore up to 50% HTx centres worldwide are using a protocol with high IS for the early post-operative period (=Induction therapy or augmented IS therapy) [12].

Interactions of IS drugs and other medications may be extensively and categorised in minor, moderate and major interactions. Here only the most important and major interactions will be mentioned.

3.1 Polyclonal antibodies

Polyclonal Antibodies are derived mainly from rabbits or horses, after the animals have been immunized with human lymphocytes (ALS) or thymocytes (ATG). Polyclonal antibodies have multiple distinct antigen-combining sites resulting in the depletion of circulating T-cells, apoptosis of activated T cells and modulation of cell surface receptor molecules. The IS potential of heterologous antibodies has been demonstrated early [15] and the first clinical use of an antilymphocyte glogulin (ALG) is reported by Starzel in 1967 [16]. The heavily contamination with anti-red cells and anti-platelet antibodies was resolved by the use of human thymocytes as the antigen source, resulting in antithymocyte globulin (ATG). First studied in renal transplantation, ATG was established as fix part in the Stanford protocol for HTx [8]. They used rabbit ATG intramusculary for the first three days after HTx and then every other day. The goal was a reduction of T cells to less than 5% in peripheral blood sample.

Polyclonal Antibodies have strong IS effect but its use is limited by the production of human antibodies against the xenogeny protein fraction allowing only a short term of use. This also explains the need for corticosteroids and the use of histamine antagonist therapy to reduce the rates of anaphylactic shock. Antipyretic medication should be added when ATG/ALS is given as fever and shivering are some of the prominent side effects. Further side effects are thrombocytopenia, leucocytopenia and anemia due to antibody cross reactions. The rate of opportunistic infections might be as high as 30%. It should be administered intravenously using a dialysis catheter or a central venous access. When administered intravenously using a peripheral vein, phlebitis may result and when given intramuscular local painful swelling leading to an abcess can occur. The goals of use of ATG/ALS in modern IS protocols are: Reducing or even avoiding CNIs due to their nephrotoxic side effects for the first days after HTx establishing a CNI free induction therapy, avoiding under-immunosuppression in the first postoperative days and treating acute cellular rejections when other regimes fail. Monitoring of polyclonal antibody treatment is difficult as the effectiveness might vary from charge to charge. Monitoring was done by achieving leucopenia later followed by using the rosette test [18]; nowadays the fluorescence activated cell sorter (FACS) analyses and T cell counts may be used. Most centres use a fixe dose regime.

3.2 Anti-Interleuckin 2 receptor antibodies

Agents who specific block the interleukin 2 (IL-2) receptor on activated T-cells, were developed to be more effective compared to non-selective polyclonal or monoclonal antibodies. An activated IL-2 receptor leads to rapid T cells proliferation and finally to the activation of B cells resulting in the production of antibodies against the allograft. The IL-2 receptor consists of three transmembrane protein chains: α (CD25), β (CD122), and γ (CD132). Basiliximab (trade name Simulect) and daclizumab (trade name Zenapax) are humanized antibodies produced by recombinant DNA technology; both composite of about human (90%) and murine (10%) antibody sequences. They are derivate from non-human species and are monoclonal antibodies to the alpha (CD 25) subunit of the IL-2 receptor. The subunit where the IL-2 receptor blocker binds to is only expressed on activated but not on resting lymphocytes. Both drugs were first used in renal transplantation and are now increasingly used in HTx recipients either as induction therapy or for the treatment of graft rejection. FDA approval for dacluzimab was in 1997 and for basiliximab in 1998. Both drugs are given intravenously and should be given within 2 to 24 hours after transplantation. Repetition should be done within 4 days (basiliximab) or 2 weeks (daclizumab). Due to the different half life time of the agents: 7.2 days for basiliximab and 20 days for daclizumab. Serum levels may be measured by ELISA and are recommended for basiliximab 0.2 ug/ml (about 20mg two times in four days) and for daclizumab 5 to 10 ug/ml to achieve a proper saturation of the receptors. When given 2.5 to 25 mg of basiliximab twice (day 0 and 4) approximately 90% of available IL-2 receptors on T lymphocytes are blocked. Saturation maintained with basiliximab for 4 to 6 weeks, with daclizumab for about 90 to 120 days. It was shown that anti-IL-2 receptor antibodies when combined with standard triple druge regime for induction therapy compared to placebo reduces rejection episodes [19, 20]. In a trial using daclizumab 1 mg per kg within 24 hours after HTx and repeated every two weeks for a total dosage of five, less rejection rates compared to placebo were seen [19]. In a later study it was shown that two doses of daclizumab are similar effective in preventing rejection as five doses, with no negative effects on patient survival [21]. Specific blockade of IL-2 receptor may prevent rejection without inducing global immunosuppression; but even if in the initial studies no increased opportunistic infections rates were observed alike to all IS agents increased risk of infection is still present. Similar to polyclonal antibodies allergic reactions are serious side effects. Anti-IL-2 receptor antibodies are only part of a multiple drug regime. There is a higher risk of lymphoma. Other side effects like nausea, vomiting, diarrhea, tremor, insomnia, headache, tremors, flu symptoms or swelling of peripheral tissue have been reported. A cytocine release syndrome has been reported as well. If anti-IL-2 receptor antibodies are as effective as polyclonal antibodies is still controversial [22, 23].

3.3 Calcineurin inhibitors

Calcineurin (CN) is an enzyme dephosphorylating the nuclear factor of activated T-cells complex (NF-ATC) which is in charge for the transcription promotor of Interleukin 2 (IL-2) production. CN is activated when an antigen-presenting cell interacts with a T cell receptor leading to an up-regulation of IL-2 production. IL-2 itself activates T-helper lymphocytes and stimulates the production of cytokines [24]. It is discussed that the absolute amount of produced IL-2 influences the extent of the immune system. Drugs blocking CN are named Calcineurin Inhibitors (CNIs); Cyclosporine A (CsA) and Tacrolimus (TAC) are the most prominent agents out of this group. For all CNIs nephrotoxic and neurologic side effects are an issue and dose reduction or even avoidance of CNIs in HTx protocols have been studied extensively. Nevertheless CNIs are still a major part of IS therapy after HTx.

3.3.1 Cyclosporine A

Cyclosporine A (CsA) is a lipophil, cyclic polypeptide consisting of 11 amino acids. It binds to cyclophylin (CpN), forming a complex which blocks C, resulting it, resulting in a suppression of activated T-cells and B-cell function. In 1971 CsA was isolated from the fungus Tolypocladium inflatum, found at the Hardanger Vidda in Norway. It was first investigated as anti-fungal antibiotic but the antibiotic spectrum was too narrow for clinical use. Its immunosuppressive activity found in 1972 was first reported in 1976 by Borel [25]. Thereafter the effectiveness in animal and human studies was investigated by Calne and his group in Cambridge [26]. They soon discovered that CsA improved heterogenic heart allografts in rats [27]. The effectiveness of CsA was confirmed in human studies in the filed of renal transplantation reported by Calne [28, 29]. These studies already recognizing the disadvantages of CsA, like the high rate of lymphoma [28] and its nephrotoxic side effects [30, 31]. It was the Stanford group who introduced CsA into clinical practice for HTx [17]. After animal research with heterotopic and orthotopic HTx in monkey, they introduced CsA to 66 patients and achieved a one year survival of 80%. At that time the starting dose of CsA was 18mg/kg per day combined with AzA and corticosteroids. European countries followed this protocol [32, 33]. Today when starting CsA recommended dosages are: intravenously (i.v.) application: either 2 to 4 mg/kg once a day continuous over 24 hours or over 4 to 6 hours, 1 to 2 mg/kg twice a day over 4 to 6 hours; oral application: 8 to 12 mg/kg/day in 2 divided doses is common. Afterwards dosage is adjusted to target trough levels and dosage reduction is aimed as low as 3 to 5 mg/kg/day.

When CsA is given per oral it is resorbed in the upper intestinal tract 30 to 60 minutes after the drug intake. The resorption is influenced by ingestion especially by grapefruit juice. The resoprtion half time is about 60 minutes. CsA is metabolized by the p450-3A enzyme in the intestinal wall epithelium. After passing the portal blood stream only 30% of the original CsA suspension will be in the systemic blood stream. The first commercially available oral formulation was very variable on absorption and blood concentration and it was tried to overcome this effect [34]. At the beginning of the 1990ies a new Cyclosporine microemulsion (Sandimmun Neoral, Novartis, Basel, Switzerland) was developed, resulting in a higher bioavailability and reducing the individual deviation attributed to ingestion. The new suspension reaches the maximum blood concentration after 1.5 to 2 hours [35, 36]. CsA is lipophil and the highest concentrations are found in the adipose tissue and in the liver. It is eliminated with a mean half time of 6 to 8 hours mainly across the liver, only 6% across the kidney. Elimination half time in children and lower in women or patients with chronic liver disease [37].

When CsA was introduced to clinical practice the rejection monitoring and drug monitoring was at its beginning. Clinical practice rejection monitoring was done by series of ECG to see voltage drops. Drug monitoring was done by the toxic side effect of AzA, monitoring the absolute T-cell number to see a severe depression. None of these methods were practicable for CsA monitoring as it is not affecting the T cell count. It became clear that a better monitoring of drug availability and a better monitoring of rejection episodes are necessary. The introduction of endomyocardial biopsy (EMB) made histologic examination possible [38]. CsA treatment and rejection monitoring with EMB resulted in a significant reduction of rejection episodes but incidence of malignant lymphoma and early renal dysfunction increased drastically [17, 28, 29, 39]. Measurement of CsA concentration in the blood stream was initiated; at first hindered as there are over 20 metabolits of CsA and the concentration itself in the blood stream is low. Today tow different methods are used for CsA measurement: In clinical practice the immunoassay (IA) is the most practicable. Different IAs have been introduced, like the radioimmunoassy, enzyme-multiplied immunoassay and florescence-polarisations immunoassay; all are using antibodies to CsA. The more specific method is the high-performance liquid chromatography (HPLC) which may be combined with mass spectrometry (MS). Measuring CsA concentration may be done before the patient takes the drug (pre-dose level, C0 measrument) or 2 hours after the intake of the drug (C2 measurement, 2 hours post dose). The C0 level is the more frequent and commonly used measurement but the C2 shows better correlation with the area under the curve and acute rejection episodes. A better prediction of long-term graft survival by C2 measurement was reported as well [40].

Finding the optimal dose and blood level for CsA treatment was and is still a challenge. The The initial Stanford protocol included ATG, corticosteroids and CsA with an initial dose of 18mg/kg followed by 10mg/kg per day [7]. The protocol was modified and CsA was adapted to the measurements of CsA blood trough levels, using a target area of 100 to 300 ng/ml, followed by a further decrease to 100 to 300 ng/ml for the first month and then lowered to 50 to 150 ng/ml in combination with AzA and ATG (for the first 7 days after HTx). This trend of avoiding high dosage of CsA to reduce the incidence of lymphoma and avoid CNI-induced nephrotoxicity has not ended yet. With the introduction of Everolimus a further dosage reduction of CsA without losing effectiveness was possible [41, 42].

Co-administration with CsA will increase serum levels of HMG-CoA reductase-inhibitors, strong inhibitors of CYP450-3A4 significantly increase the blood concentrations of CsA. Sulfonamides, rifampin and carbamacepine reduce CsA concentrations.

3.3.2 Tacrolimus

Tacrolimus (TAC) blocks the CN by forming a complex with the FK506 binding protein resulting in the suppression of T-lymphocyte activation and cytokine production (IL2, 3 , 4, Interferon and tumor necrosis factor [TNF]). The structure of the macrolide antibiotic isolated from Streptomyces tsukubaensis is more similar to Rapamycin than to CsA. TAC was described seven years after the introduction of CsA [10] and found to be 100 times more potent [43]. It was first clinical used in 10 HTx recipients at the University of Pittsburgh in combination with steroids [44, 45]. When given per oral its absorption half-life is about 5 to 6 hours and the bioavailability is about 20%, depending on the intake of food (fat food reduces the bioavailability, grapefruit juice increases the blood concentration); it is mainly absorbed in the duodenum and jejunum, far less in the ileum and colon. 75 - 99% bind to proteins and the elimination half-life is 11.7 hours. Its bioavailability is higher in patients with impaired liver function. TAC has a large inter- and intraindividual variation in the pharmacokinetics. Extraction is mainly through the stool and it can not be removed by dialysis. Similar to CsA TAC should be given in two divided dose every 12 hours starting orally with 0.1 to 0.3 mg/kg/day, intravenously 0.01-0.03 mg/kg/day. Intravenously dosage in pediatric HTx might be raised up to 0.03 to 0.05 mg/kg/day.

Monitoring of the trough level is commercially done by an enzyme-linked immunosorbent assay (ELISA) or microparticulate enzyme immunoassay. Drug interactions are similar to CsA (inhibitor or inducers of P4503A4 may alter TAC level).

TAC seems to reduce the numbers of rejection episodes compared to CsA; in 1992 an actuarial freedom from rejection in the TAC group at 90 days after HTx of 41% and 28% of recurrent rejection was reported [44]. Especially in children TAC is increasingly used [46].

Until recently TAC was marked as Prograf (Astellas Pharma US, Inc., Deerfield, IL) and had to be taken twice a day similar to CsA (Sandimune Neoral, Novartis Pharmaceuticals, Basel, Switzerland); now a retard drug was released named Advagraf (Astellas Pharma US, Inc., Deerfield, IL), which may be taken just once a day. It was studied in renal and liver transplant patients; approval for HTx is investigated.

Even if very close related to CsA there are clinical relevant differences especially regarding side effects of the drug. TAC has a higher incidence of de-novo diabetes mellitus, a higher rate of anaemia and is increasing the tonus of the muscle. CsA on the other side leads to gingival hyperplasia, arterial hypertension, hirsuitsm, and increases liver laboratory values.

3.4 Purine synthesis inhibitors

Purine synthesis inhibitors (also called Antimetabolites) can halt cell growth and cell division either in a very unselective way (Azathiporine, [AzA]) or a more specific way (Mycophenolate Mofetil, Enteric-coated mycophenolate mofetil). Since the beginning of modern transplantation medicine purine synthesis inhibitors (AzA) have been part of the IS protocol. Between 2000 and 2009 the reported use of purine synthesis inhibitors to the international registry for heart and lung transplantation (International Society for Heart and Lung Transplantation, ISHLT) as maintenance therapy in HTx recipients was over 85% [12].

3.4.1 Azathioprine

The pro-drug of 6-Mercaptopurin, a thiopurin substance, called Azathioprine (AzA) is a purine analogue IS drug which has antiproliverative effects especially on fast growing cells; i.e. T-cells and B-cells. AzA is metabolized to 6-Mercaptopurin which is less effective [47, 48]. AzA blocks the mitosis of cells resulting in an inhibition of proliferation of activated T and B lymphocytes and it seems that AzA is blocking the production of IL2 too. Nevertheless its complete mechanism of action is still not fully understood. The antiprolivaertive effect is not limited to T and B cells but also on bone marrow, hepatic or other cells. This leads to its severe side effects: bone marrow depression resulting in leucopenia and thrombocytopenia and its hepatotoxic side effects. Other side effects like nausea, vomiting or diarrhoea have been reported mainly at higher doses. Long term treatment might be associated with acute pancreatitis.

AzA was one of the first drugs used to prevent allograft rejection and its first human use in HTx was reported by the Stanford group [49]. The Standford protocol used AzA 1.5-2.5 mg/kg per day combined with corticosteroids. Today starting dosage recommendations is once a day 3 to 5 mg/kg orally or i.v. and may be reduced to 1 to 3mg/kg as maintenance therapy.

Its peak plasma concentration is reached within 1 to 2 hours after oral intake and its plasma half-life time is 3 to 6 hours. AzA is eliminated mainly by the kidney.

One of the weak points of AzA treatment is the unspecific monitoring. Daily dosage administration is still adapted depending on the toxic side effects trying to target the white blood cell count between 4000mm^3 and 6000mm^3. Lately there are reports of monitoring AzA treatment by blood concentrations of 6-thioguanin [50]. When AzA is combined with allopurinol the dose should be reduced to 75% to avoid severe pancytopenia as allopurinol affects the metabolism of 6-Mercaptopurine. AzA may reduce the anticoagulant effect of Warfarin [51].

AzA had a major positive impact on post-transplant outcome but due to its unspecific way of action, severe side effects and the disadvantage of specific monitoring AzA was replaced in many IS protocols. On the other hand it is increasingly used in evolving countries due to its lower costs.

3.4.2 Mycophenolic acid

Mycophenolic acid (MPA) is the activated IS species of mycophenolate mofetil (MMF). MPA is derived from the fungus Penicillium stoloniferum and was marked as MMF. To improve its bioavailability mycophenolate sodium was developed (see 3.4.2.1). MMF is a dehydrogenase controlling the synthesis rate of guanine monophosphate resulting in an inhibition of purines. Compared to AzA it specifically suppresses proliferation of T and B lymphocytes without severe bone marrow depression. In large multicentre trails the superiority of MMF over AZA was reported resulting in a progressively replacement of AzA by MMF [2,52,53,54].

Following oral administration it is rapidly metabolised 100% to MPA in the intestinal tract and the liver. No plasma MMF concentration will be measured in the blood, only MPA. MPA is bound 97% to albumin and metabolized in the liver and intestinal tract to a stable phenolic glucuronide (MPAG) which is not pharmacologically active. The maximum plasma concentration of MPA is reached about 1 hour after oral intake and its half-life time is around 16 hours (the same is true for MPAG). Over 90% of MPA is extracted by the kidney but MPAG is extracted by the bile. MPAG enters the enterohepatic cycling process; it is metabolised in the intestinal tract back to MPA and reabsorbed. This leads to a second peak in the plasma concentration after 6 to 12 hours of intake. No dosage adjustment in patient with renal impairment or haemodialysis is needed. In patients with a reduced glomerular filtration rate (GFR) a 3-to 6-fold higher MPAG area under the curve values were reported [55, 56]. In combination with TAC a 50% lower dose of MMF compared to a combination with CsA is recommended as CsA inhibits the hepatic extraction of MPAG leading to a reduced rate of enterohepatic recirculation. . MPA/MPAG can not be removed by hemodialysis. Side effects of MMF are vomiting, diarrhoea and other gastrointestinal side effects [57]. Diabetes and necrosis of bones have been related to MMF. A study were MMF was tested in pediatric HTx recipients showed that genetic polymorphism can directly Influence adverse events of MMF [58].

Initial trials using MMF used standard dosage of 1g in combination with CsA and did not use therapeutic drug monitoring; today dosage recommendation is 1g to 1.5 g twice a day orally or i.v. but when given i.v. dosage shoulkd be given at least over two hours.

Due to the complex pharmacokinetics of MPA and not adequately reflected MPA trough concentrations when combined with TAC, drug level measurement of MPA is still not widely common. HPLC with ultraviolet detection and mass spectrometric may be used to measure free MPA concentrations. Some centres describe the use of an enzyme-multiplied immunoassay technique. Simultaneouse application of acyclovir, ganciclovir and high doses of salicylates are enhancing plasma concentrations of MPAG; antacids, colestyramin and CsA are lowering it. To reduce the gastrointestinal side effects of MMF it was coated (see 3.4.2.1).

3.4.2.1 Enteric-coated Mycophenolate sodium

Enteric-coated Mycophenolate sodiumfortic (EC-MPS) is an enterie formulation of mycophenolate sodium (a prodrug of MPA). MPA reversible inhibits the inosine monophosphate dehydrogenase and the pathway of guanosine nucleotide synthesis which affects B and T lymphocytes whereas other cell types can utilize salvage pathyways for purine synthesis. The coating of mycophenolate sodium should reduce the gastrointestinal side effects [59]. In renal transplant recipients a dosage of 720 mg EC-MPS twice a day was therapeutically equivalent to MMF 1000 mg twice a day with comparable safety profile [60].

Dosage recommendation in HTx recipients is 720mg twice a day either orally or intravenously. Optimal measurement of EC-MPS plasma concentration due to its delay in reaching maximal blood concentrations compared to MMF, is yet not clarify (C0, C2, C4, C6).

3.5 Proliferation signal inhibitors

Proliferation signal Inhibitors (PSI) (also named mammalian target of rapamycin (mTOR) inhibitors) include two important drugs currently available for organ transplantation: Rapamycin (Rapa) or Sirolimus (SRL) and Everolimus (EvE). Four decades ago Rapa was extracted and its antifungal effects reported [61]. Intensive research resulted in the discovery of the target of rapamycin named mTOR. mTOR is a serine-threonine kinase which is a transducer of information from growth factors and energy sensors within the cell. Both drugs form a complex with the intracellular binding protein FKBP-12, (similar to FK 506) but contrarily to TAC the PSIs inhibit the activity of mTOR. This leads to an arrest of a cell cycle in the mid-to-late G1 phase [61, 62]. While FK 506 is suppressing lymphokine production and blocking activation of T-cells, PSIs inhibit cells proliferation by impairing their response to growth-promoting lymphokines [63, 64]. They are also used in other areas of medicine like oncology or interventional cardiology (drug eluting stents).

3.5.1 Rapamycin

Rapamycin (Rapa) is a macrocyclic lactone with antifungal, antibiotic and IS properties. It was discovered in 1965, extracted out of soil taken from Rapa Nui in New Zeeland [65]. Its IS effects were discovered in the 1990s [61]. During the approval studies for Rapa the anti-tumor effects of Rapa and its analogues like EvE were found introducing them in oncology and for the prevention of restenosis after percutaneous coronary angioplasty.

Rapa has structural similarities to FK 506 binding protein but it forms complex with FKBP12 which results in an inhibitor of the mTOR [66]. This leads to suppression of T and B cells and decreases the population of dentritic cells who present antigen to T cells during activation [67].

The bioavailability of Rapa is 20% and decreases with food rich in fats (see 3.5.2); 92% of Rapa binds to albumin, is metabolism extensively in intestinal wall via p-glycoprotein and in the liver by CYP3A4. Seven major metabolites are known but 90% of the IS activity is done by Rapa; close to 90% is eliminated by the liver only 2% by the kidney. In contrast to EvE half-life time of Rapa is about 62 hours ± 16 hours allowing one single daily dose.

A loading dose for Rapa on the first post-transplantation day is recommended; in renal transplantation the loading dose should be 3 times the estimated maintenance dose (normally 2mg), in HTx recipients 15mg are given followed by a maintenance dose of 5mg and further guided by trough levels. The total dosage must no exceed 40mg per day; if a higher dose is needed it should be divided over a period of 2 days. In children with a body weight below 40 kg initially a loading dose of 3mg/m^2 and a maintenance dose of 1mg/m^2 daily is recommended. If CNI therapy is reduced, Rapa dosage should be increased according to the targeted trough levels. In patient with severe hepatic impairment Rapa dosage should be reduced.

Routine clinical measurement is done with chromatographic methods. Major side effects of Rapa are swelling in different tissues, prolonging healing of wounds, increasing cholesterol and triglyceride levels, proteinuria as well as blood pressure. Rapa induced interstitial lung disease like pneumonitis have been observed [68-70]. When combined with CNIs, CNIs dosage reduction is necessary otherwise worsening renal function will develop. Rapa recommended blood trough levels in combination with CNIs is between 4 to 12 ng/ml, without CsA a four times higher Rapa dosage might be needed (CsA/CNIs suppress the metebolizion of Rapa), the recommended blood trough levels is increased between 12 to 20 Ng/ml depending on the time after transplantation. This is also the reason why Rapa intake when combined with CNIs is recommended four hours after CNI administration. Otherwise Rapa enhance the toxic effect of CNIs with an increased risk of CNI induced hemolytic uremic syndrome, thrombotic thrombocytopenic purpura and thrombotic microangiogiopathy. Drugs inducing CYP3A4 (Rifampicin) will decrease, strong inhibitors (Macrolides, Ketoconazole, Itraconazole) will increase Rapa blood levels. Similarly to CNIs grapefruit juice increases plasma concentration of Rapa. According to the last ISHLT report Rapa is currently used up to 20 % of HTx recipients [12].

3.5.2 Everolimus

Everolimus (EvE) is an analogue of Rapa and differs only by one extra hydroxyethyl group at position 40; still this leads to some differences. EvE blocks growth factor-mediated proliferation of cells including vascular smooth muscle cell through a CA2+ independent signal [71]. Following oral intakc EvE is rapidly absorbed and reaches its maximal blood concentrations after 1 to 2 hours. The oral bioavailability is approximately 30% [72-75] and it is altered by food; a high-fat meal is slowing down the absorption of EvE. It is recommended that EvE is taken constantly either with or without food. EvE undergoes major metabolism with none of the metabolites reaching significantly IS activity. Its half-life time is 28 hours and compared to Rapa (62 hours) much shorter. Initial dose may be 0.75 mg twice a day, no loading dose is necessary.

EvE has a more rapid time to steady state compared to Rapa (4 versus 6 days). EvE binds to plasma proteins about 75% to 80% and is mainly eliminated in the liver, only 5% are extracted across the kidney. In patient with severe hepatic impairment EvE dosage should be reduced. PSIs and CNIs are metabolised by cytochrome P4503A4 (CYP3A4) isoenzyme leading to reduced clearance of EvE when CNI is given. Pre-clinical research reported of no nephrotoxicity of EvE [76] but when it was first clinical used combined with full dose CsA it showed worsening renal function [77, 78]. For that reason FDA approval was refused, but the European Medicine Agency (EMEA) approved EvE for further studies. In a prospective multicentre study the possibility of dose reduction of CsA combined with EvE resulted in stable renal function without loss of efficacy [79]. Further trials confirmed this [41, 42, 80]. Besides this interaction drugs who strong induce CYP3A4 will decrease, strong inhibitors will increase EvE blood levels. Reported EvE blood trough levels are within 3 to 8 ng/ml. Drug monitoring is done by HPLC coupled with mass spectrometry and an immunoassay is being developed. EvE showed to have antiproliferative effects delaying the onset of cardiac transplant vasculopathy and reducing the rate of CMV infections [77, 81]; it is increasingly used, up to 2.6 % in HTx recipients in the years 2008 and 2009 [12]. Due to the favourable effects it may be used in children and is currently investigated (RAD 2313).

3.6 Immunosuppressive regimes

At the beginning little was know about interaction, side-effects and combination of IS drugs. Nowadays with many different IS drugs acting at different receptors and stages of the immune system more effective and less toxic regimes may be used.

It was revealed that the combination of different acting IS drugs with adjusted dosage enhance their effectiveness and reduce toxicity. To avoid nephrotoxic side effects of CNIs and to achieve a high IS, over 50% of the centres reporting to the ISHLT are using an induction therapy (20% using polyclonal antibodies, 30% use IL2 receptor antibodies) [12]. Conventionally for maintenance therapy patients are treated with a triple drug regimens, consisting of a CNI (CyC, TAC), antiproliferative agent (AzA, MMF) and corticosteroids. Shortly after the introduction of CsA in 1980 Griffith and colleagues used CsA in combination with low-dose steroids in HTx recipients, tapering steroids from 200mg per day to 15 mg per day similar to the regime used by Starzel in renal and liver transplant recipients [82-84]. Combining CsA, AzA and Cortocosteroides, commonly called triple-drug immunsupression, evolved and showed improved survival for short, medium and long term follow-up [85, 86]. It increased 1 years survival after HTx from 60% to 80% and became the standard regime not only in the US but also in European countries over the next 30 years [87, 88]. The triple-drug protocol, even if modified (many centres skipping corticosteroids after a certain time) is still used around the globe. Adding a forth drug to the regime has been reported but became not standard [19, 89].

Still due to the well know side effects of IS, associated with a significant morbidity, discussion about reducing IS will continue. Reduce IS therapy with a mono or dual drug regimes are investigated. Recently a retrospective study involving 150 patients within 28 days after HTx maintaining recipients only on monotherapy with TAC has been published [90]. One has to notice that in IS monotherapy compliance is paramount and could result in a disastrous outcome. The conviction of currently experts in the field of IS is, that today's "standard" immunosuppression may be replaced by IS individualized for each patient on the basis of genomic profile, baseline risks for rejection and infection, and perhaps serial assessments of immune response after transplantation [91].

4. Immunosuppression for acute rejection

Different principles of IS treatment after organ transplantation have been established over time. After HTx numbers of rejection episodes and immune reactivity are highest within the first 3-6 months. Therefore one of the principles is to use the highest intensity of IS immediately after surgery and decrease it over the first year (Induction therapy (see 3.1), corticosteroid weaning (see 4.1.2); lowering blood concentrations of IS agents). The second principle is to rather admit more IS drugs with non-overlapping toxic side effects at a low dose rather than a higher and more toxic dose of a single drug. Therefore monitoring of the IS drug trough levels is of great interest; special caution must be paid to interaction of the drugs (lowering or increasing the blood levels) or i.e. diarrhea when orally taken. The goal is to avoid over-immunosuppression, which leads to infection and malignancy. This on the other hand may lead to late acute rejection episodes even if it is rare [92]. Corner stone of the treatment are corticosteroids, both oral or intravenous, ATG (see 3.1 Polyclonal Antibodies),

IL-2 receptor blockers (see 3.2 Interleukin 2 receptor antibodies) or murine monoclonal antibody (see 4.2). The type of treatment depends on clinical status of the recipients (if the rejection is hemodynamic compromising [reduced cardiac output, decreased pulmonary artery saturation, elevated wedge pressure, reduced cardiac index]) the histology degree and severity of the rejection. Moderate to severe rejection episodes need therapy: intravenous corticosteroids for three to five days, intensify oral maintenance IS therapy and eventually change to another protocol; if there are recurrent rejection episodes TAC or EvE may be considered. In patients with hemodynamic impairment additionally polyclonal or monoclonal antibodies or plasmapheresis should be kept in mind.

4.1 Corticosteroids

Corticosteroids inhibit the synthesis of cytokines, but the exact mechanism of action in solving acute rejection is not jet completely understood. Steroids suppress besides i.e. IL-6, interferon gamma, TNF, the production of IL-1 resulting in a diminished production of IL-2 by activated T cells. In animal models it was reported that steroids induce lymphocytolysis which was not proved in humans. Synthetic pharmaceutical drugs with corticosteroid-like effect are used in a variety of treatments. Prednisone is the most used synthetic steroid and is five times more potent compared to cortisol. Its bioavailability is 70% when orally taken and it is metabolised in the liver. Natural steroid hormones have a very short half-life time, synthetic steroids like prednisone have a half-life time of 1 hour. The side effects of long-term corticosteroids are commonly known; dosage reduction below the cushing threshold or even weaning them off are valid options. Nevertheless for acute rejection episodes intravenously high dose corticosteroid treatment is still necessary and effective. After solving the acute phase of the rejection episode orally corticosteroids should be introduced to treatment for at least some time or if already part of the maintenance IS protocol its dosage should be increased.

4.1.2 Corticodsteroid weaning

Over 85% of the centres reporting to the ISHLT are currently using corticosteroids within the first year after HTx, after 5 years about 50% are still using corticosteroids [12, 46]. The negative side effects of steroids are well known such as i.e. weight gain, glucose intolerance, dyslipidemia, osteoporosis, or cartaract. Most of the rejection episodes are within the first year after HTx and most of the steroids can be taken off over a course of a few months. The rationale, for diminishing the overall use of corticosteroids is the availability of new IS agents acting more selective compared to synthetic corticosteroids. Numerous protocols were established, most of them use a high dosage of corticosteroids intra-operative (when starting reperfusion) and within the first days (as part of an induction therapy). When oral dosage is given different possibilities are available such as i.e. fixed dose of 15 mg per day or prednisolon 0.05 to 2mg/kg divided by one to four doses per day. After weeks of months the dose is reduced achieving a dose below the cushing threshold. Some study groups report to take off corticosteroids as early as 8 weeks after HTx [90] or over a course for several months following a simple weaning protocol guided by daily cortisol measurments to avoid onset of adrenal insufficiency (level > 8 µg/dl continue to wean, otherwise continue steroid therapy) (Baran DA. A prospective trial of steroid discontinuation in stable heart transplant patients as guided by serum cortisol measurement. International Society for Heart and Lung Transplantation 2009, Abstract 431). Other weaning protocols decrese the daily prednisone dosage by 1mg each month starting at month 6 post HTx [93].

The question why long-term use of corticosteroids is still that present may have several reasons i.e. avoiding adrenal insufficiency or other potential effects when treatment is stopped but also the 'heritage' of this therapy as steroids once were nearly the only immunosuppressant choice for transplant recipients.

4.2 Monoclonal muromonab CD3 antibody

Muromonab-CD3 (brand name: OKT3) is a monoclonal antibody against CD3 antigen resulting in an inhibition of T-cell function by down regulation of CD3 positive cells. It was the first monoclonal antibody to be approved for clinical use in humans. Similar to polyclonal antibodies its way of administration is only intravenously. Recommended dosage is 5 mg per day, in pediatric patients (< 30kg body weight) initial dosage may be lowered to 2.5mg per day. The human body will produce human anti-mice antibodies, as OKT3 is like a mice-antibody explaining the loss of effectivity if given repeatedly. Toxic side effects besides the well know from all IS agents (higher infection rate higher rate of lymphoproliferative disorders) have been reported: cytokine-mediated first-dose reaction, pulmonary edema, aseptic meningitis, haemolytic-uremic syndrome. The first-dose reaction may include fever, rigors, nausea, vomiting, and diarrhea which will decrease with repeated exposure. Nevertheless steroids, antihistamines and antipyretics should be given along with OKT3 to minimize these side effects. It takes about a week after ending the OKT3 treatment until the T cell function returns to normal.

5. References

[1] Dutkowski P, de Rougemont O, Clavien PA. Alexis Carrel: genius, innovator and ideologist. Am J Transplant. 2008 Oct;8(10):1998-2003.

[2] Mathew TH. A blinded, long-term, randomized multicenter study of mycophenolate mofetil in cadaveric renal transplantation: results at three years. Tricontinental Mycophenolate Mofetil Renal Transplantation Study Group. Transplantation. 1998 Jun 15;65(11):1450-4.

[3] Lower RR, Shumway NE. Studies on orthotopic homotransplantation of the canine heart. Surgical forum. 1960;11:18-9.

[4] Shumway NE. Cardiac transplantation. The Heart bulletin. 1963 May-Jun;12:57-60.

[5] Shumway NE. Transplantation of the Heart. Surgery, gynecology & obstetrics. 1963 Sep;117:361-2.

[6] Barnard CN. Human cardiac transplantation. An evaluation of the first two operations performed at the Groote Schuur Hospital, Cape Town. The American journal of cardiology. 1968 Oct;22(4):584-96.

[7] Wallwork J. Heart and heart-lung transplantation. Philadelphia: Saunders 1989.

[8] Bieber CP, Griepp RB, Oyer PE, Wong J, Stinson EB. Use of rabbit antithymocyte globulin in cardiac transplantation. Relationship of serum clearance rates to clinical outcome. Transplantation. 1976 Nov;22(5):478-88.

[9] Calne RY, White DJ, Thiru S, Evans DB, McMaster P, Dunn DC, et al. Cyclosporin A in patients receiving renal allografts from cadaver donors. Lancet. 1978 Dec 23-30;2(8104-5):1323-7.

[10] Kino T, Hatanaka H, Miyata S, Inamura N, Nishiyama M, Yajima T, et al. FK-506, a novel immunosuppressant isolated from a Streptomyces. II. Immunosuppressive effect of FK-506 in vitro. The Journal of antibiotics. 1987 Sep;40(9):1256-65.

[11] Starzl TE, Todo S, Fung J, Demetris AJ, Venkataramman R, Jain A. FK 506 for liver, kidney, and pancreas transplantation. Lancet. 1989 Oct 28;2(8670):1000-4.

[12] Stehlik J, Edwards LB, Kucheryavaya AY, Aurora P, Christie JD, Kirk R, et al. The Registry of the International Society for Heart and Lung Transplantation: twenty-seventh official adult heart transplant report--2010. J Heart Lung Transplant. Oct;29(10):1089-103.

[13] Brewin TB, Cole MP, Jones CT, Platt DS, Todd ID. Mycophenolic acid (NSC-129185): preliminary clinical trials. Cancer chemotherapy reports. 1972 Feb;56(1):83-7.

[14] Morris RE, Hoyt EG, Murphy MP, Eugui EM, Allison AC. Mycophenolic acid morpholinoethylester (RS-61443) is a new immunosuppressant that prevents and halts heart allograft rejection by selective inhibition of T- and B-cell purine synthesis. Transplantation proceedings. 1990 Aug;22(4):1659-62.

[15] Woodruff MF, Symes MO, Anderson NF. The Effect of Intraperitoneal Injection of Thoracic Duct Lymphocytes from Normal and Immunized Rats in Mice Inoculated with the Landschutz Ascites Tumour. British journal of cancer. 1963 Sep;17:482-7.

[16] Starzl TE, Marchioro TL, Porter KA, Iwasaki Y, Cerilli GJ. The use of heterologous antilymphoid agents in canine renal and liver homotransplantation and in human renal homotransplantation. Surgery, gynecology & obstetrics. 1967 Feb;124(2):301-8.

[17] Oyer PE. Heart transplantation in the cyclosporine era. The Annals of thoracic surgery. 1988 Nov;46(5):489-90.

[18] Bach MA, Bach JF. Studies on thymus products. VI. The effects of cyclic nucleotides and prostaglandins on rosette-forming cells. Interactions with thymic factor. European journal of immunology. 1973 Dec;3(12):778-83.

[19] Beniaminovitz A, Itescu S, Lietz K, Donovan M, Burke EM, Groff BD, et al. Prevention of rejection in cardiac transplantation by blockade of the interleukin-2 receptor with a monoclonal antibody. The New England journal of medicine. 2000 Mar 2;342(9):613-9.

[20] Nashan B, Moore R, Amlot P, Schmidt AG, Abeywickrama K, Soulillou JP. Randomised trial of basiliximab versus placebo for control of acute cellular rejection in renal allograft recipients. CHIB 201 International Study Group. Lancet. 1997 Oct 25;350(9086):1193-8.

[21] Ortiz V, Almenar L, Martinez-Dolz L, Zorio E, Chamorro C, Moro J, et al. Induction therapy with daclizumab in heart transplantation--how many doses? Transplantation proceedings. 2006 Oct;38(8):2541-3.

[22] Flaman F, Zieroth S, Rao V, Ross H, Delgado DH. Basiliximab versus rabbit anti-thymocyte globulin for induction therapy in patients after heart transplantation. J Heart Lung Transplant. 2006 Nov;25(11):1358-62.
[23] Mattei MF, Redonnet M, Gandjbakhch I, Bandini AM, Billes A, Epailly E, et al. Lower risk of infectious deaths in cardiac transplant patients receiving basiliximab versus anti-thymocyte globulin as induction therapy. J Heart Lung Transplant. 2007 Jul;26(7):693-9.
[24] Yamashita M, Katsumata M, Iwashima M, Kimura M, Shimizu C, Kamata T, et al. T cell receptor-induced calcineurin activation regulates T helper type 2 cell development by modifying the interleukin 4 receptor signaling complex. The Journal of experimental medicine. 2000 Jun 5;191(11):1869-79.
[25] Borel JF, Feurer C, Gubler HU, Stahelin H. Biological effects of cyclosporin A: a new antilymphocytic agent. Agents and actions. 1976 Jul;6(4):468-75.
[26] Nagao T, White DJ, Calne RY. Kinetics of unresponsiveness induced by a short course of cyclosporin A. Transplantation. 1982 Jan;33(1):31-5.
[27] Kostakis A. Early experience with cyclosporine: a historic perspective. Transplantation proceedings. 2004 Mar;36(2 Suppl):22S-4S.
[28] Merrill JP. Publications of John P. Merrill. Nephron. 1978;22(1-3):265-80.
[29] Cyclosporin a as sole immunosuppressive agent in recipients of kidney allografts from cadaver donors. Preliminary results of a European multicentre trial. Lancet. 1982 Jul 10;2(8289):57-60.
[30] Kahan. Cyclosporine: nursing and paraprofessional aspects. Transplantation proceedings. 1983 Dec;15(4 Suppl 1-2):3109-83.
[31] Kahan BD. Cyclosporine: a revolution in transplantation. Transplantation proceedings. 1999 Feb-Mar;31(1-2A):14S-5S.
[32] Wallwork J, McGregor CG, Wells FC, Cory-Pearce R, English TA. Cyclosporin and intravenous sulphadimidine and trimethoprim therapy. Lancet. 1983 Feb 12;1(8320):366-7.
[33] Cabrol C, Gandjbakhch I, Guiraudon G, Pavie A, Villemot JP, Viars P, et al. [Heart transplantation. Our experience at the Pitie Hospital in Paris]. Bulletin de l'Academie nationale de medecine. 1982 Feb;166(2):235-50.
[34] Kovarik JM, Mueller EA, van Bree JB, Arns W, Renner E, Kutz K. Within-day consistency in cyclosporine pharmacokinetics from a microemulsion formulation in renal transplant patients. Therapeutic drug monitoring. 1994 Jun;16(3):232-7.
[35] Klauser R, Irschik H, Kletzmayr J, Sturm I, Brunner W, Woloszczuk W, et al. Neoral--a new microemulsion formula of cyclosporine A: interpatient pharmacokinetic variability in renal transplant recipients. Transplantation proceedings. 1995 Dec;27(6):3427-9.
[36] Kovarik JM, Kallay Z, Mueller EA, van Bree JB, Arns W, Renner E. Acute effect of cyclosporin on renal function following the initial changeover to a microemulsion formulation in stable kidney transplant patients. Transpl Int. 1995;8(5):335-9.

[37] Keown PA, Stiller CR, Stawecki M, Freeman D. Pharmacokinetics of cyclosporine in solid organ transplantation. Transplantation proceedings. 1986 Dec;18(6 Suppl 5):160-4.
[38] Caves PK, Stinson EB, Billingham ME, Rider AK, Shumway NE. Diagnosis of human cardiac allograft rejection by serial cardiac biopsy. The Journal of thoracic and cardiovascular surgery. 1973 Sep;66(3):461-6.
[39] Calne RY, Rolles K, White DJ, Thiru S, Evans DB, McMaster P, et al. Cyclosporin A initially as the only immunosuppressant in 34 recipients of cadaveric organs: 32 kidneys, 2 pancreases, and 2 livers. Lancet. 1979 Nov 17;2(8151):1033-6.
[40] Nemati E, Einollahi B, Taheri S, Moghani-Lankarani M, Kalantar E, Simforoosh N, et al. Cyclosporine trough (C0) and 2-hour postdose (C2) levels: which one is a predictor of graft loss? Transplantation proceedings. 2007 May;39(4):1223-4.
[41] Schweiger M, Wasler A, Prenner G, Stiegler P, Stadlbauer V, Schwarz M, et al. Everolimus and reduced cyclosporine trough levels in maintenance heart transplant recipients. Transplant immunology. 2006 Jun;16(1):46-51.
[42] Lehmkuhl HB, Mai D, Dandel M, Knosalla C, Hiemann NE, Grauhan O, et al. Observational study with everolimus (Certican) in combination with low-dose cyclosporine in de novo heart transplant recipients. J Heart Lung Transplant. 2007 Jul;26(7):700-4.
[43] Ochiai T, Nakajima K, Nagata M, Suzuki T, Asano T, Uematsu T, et al. Effect of a new immunosuppressive agent, FK 506, on heterotopic cardiac allotransplantation in the rat. Transplantation proceedings. 1987 Feb;19(1 Pt 2):1284-6.
[44] Armitage JM, Kormos RL, Morita S, Fung J, Marrone GC, Hardesty RL, et al. Clinical trial of FK 506 immunosuppression in adult cardiac transplantation. The Annals of thoracic surgery. 1992 Aug;54(2):205-10; discussion 10-1.
[45] Armitage JM, Kormos RL, Fung J, Starzl TE. The clinical trial of FK 506 as primary and rescue immunosuppression in adult cardiac transplantation. Transplantation proceedings. 1991 Dec;23(6):3054-7.
[46] Kirk R, Edwards LB, Kucheryavaya AY, Aurora P, Christie JD, Dobbels F, et al. The Registry of the International Society for Heart and Lung Transplantation: thirteenth official pediatric heart transplantation report--2010. J Heart Lung Transplant. Oct;29(10):1119-28.
[47] Bierer BE, Somers PK, Wandless TJ, Burakoff SJ, Schreiber SL. Probing immunosuppressant action with a nonnatural immunophilin ligand. Science (New York, NY. 1990 Oct 26;250(4980):556-9.
[48] Crabtree GR. Contingent genetic regulatory events in T lymphocyte activation. Science (New York, NY. 1989 Jan 20;243(4889):355-61.
[49] Oyer PE, Stinson EB, Reitz BA, Bieber CP, Jamieson SW, Shumway NE. Cardiac transplantation: 1980. Transplantation proceedings. 1981 Mar;13(1 Pt 1):199-206.
[50] Cuffari C, Hunt S, Bayless T. Utilisation of erythrocyte 6-thioguanine metabolite levels to optimise azathioprine therapy in patients with inflammatory bowel disease. Gut. 2001 May;48(5):642-6.
[51] Reynolds PD, Hunter JO. Pharmacotherapy of inflammatory bowel disease. Digestive diseases (Basel, Switzerland). 1993 Nov-Dec;11(6):334-42.

[52] Mele TS, Halloran PF. The use of mycophenolate mofetil in transplant recipients. Immunopharmacology. 2000 May;47(2-3):215-45.
[53] Sollinger HW. Mycophenolate mofetil for the prevention of acute rejection in primary cadaveric renal allograft recipients. U.S. Renal Transplant Mycophenolate Mofetil Study Group. Transplantation. 1995 Aug 15;60(3):225-32.
[54] Placebo-controlled study of mycophenolate mofetil combined with cyclosporin and corticosteroids for prevention of acute rejection. European Mycophenolate Mofetil Cooperative Study Group. Lancet. 1995 May 27;345(8961):1321-5.
[55] Bullingham RE, Nicholls AJ, Kamm BR. Clinical pharmacokinetics of mycophenolate mofetil. Clinical pharmacokinetics. 1998 Jun;34(6):429-55.
[56] Kuypers DR, Ekberg H, Grinyo J, Nashan B, Vincenti F, Snell P, et al. Mycophenolic acid exposure after administration of mycophenolate mofetil in the presence and absence of cyclosporin in renal transplant recipients. Clinical pharmacokinetics. 2009;48(5):329-41.
[57] Knight SR, Russell NK, Barcena L, Morris PJ. Mycophenolate mofetil decreases acute rejection and may improve graft survival in renal transplant recipients when compared with azathioprine: a systematic review. Transplantation. 2009 Mar 27;87(6):785-94.
[58] Ohmann EL, Burckart GJ, Brooks MM, Chen Y, Pravica V, Girnita DM, et al. Genetic polymorphisms influence mycophenolate mofetil-related adverse events in pediatric heart transplant patients. J Heart Lung Transplant. May;29(5):509-16.
[59] Reinke P, Budde K, Hugo C, Petersen P, Schnuelle P, Fricke L, et al. Reduction of Gastrointestinal Complications in Renal Graft Recipients after Conversion from Mycophenolate Mofetil to Enteric-coated Mycophenolate Sodium. Transplantation proceedings. Jun;43(5):1641-6.
[60] Salvadori M, Holzer H, de Mattos A, Sollinger H, Arns W, Oppenheimer F, et al. Enteric-coated mycophenolate sodium is therapeutically equivalent to mycophenolate mofetil in de novo renal transplant patients. Am J Transplant. 2004 Feb;4(2):231-6.
[61] Marx SO, Jayaraman T, Go LO, Marks AR. Rapamycin-FKBP inhibits cell cycle regulators of proliferation in vascular smooth muscle cells. Circ Res. 1995 Mar;76(3):412-7.
[62] Wiederrecht GJ, Sabers CJ, Brunn GJ, Martin MM, Dumont FJ, Abraham RT. Mechanism of action of rapamycin: new insights into the regulation of G1-phase progression in eukaryotic cells. Progress in cell cycle research. 1995;1:53-71.
[63] Dumont FJ, Staruch MJ, Koprak SL, Melino MR, Sigal NH. Distinct mechanisms of suppression of murine T cell activation by the related macrolides FK-506 and rapamycin. J Immunol. 1990 Jan 1;144(1):251-8.
[64] Terada N, Lucas JJ, Szepesi A, Franklin RA, Domenico J, Gelfand EW. Rapamycin blocks cell cycle progression of activated T cells prior to events characteristic of the middle to late G1 phase of the cycle. Journal of cellular physiology. 1993 Jan;154(1):7-15.

[65] Vezina C, Kudelski A, Sehgal SN. Rapamycin (AY-22,989), a new antifungal antibiotic. I. Taxonomy of the producing streptomycete and isolation of the active principle. The Journal of antibiotics. 1975 Oct;28(10):721-6.
[66] Heitman J, Movva NR, Hall MN. Targets for cell cycle arrest by the immunosuppressant rapamycin in yeast. Science (New York, NY. 1991 Aug 23;253(5022):905-9.
[67] Woltman AM, van der Kooij SW, Coffer PJ, Offringa R, Daha MR, van Kooten C. Rapamycin specifically interferes with GM-CSF signaling in human dendritic cells, leading to apoptosis via increased p27KIP1 expression. Blood. 2003 Feb 15;101(4):1439-45.
[68] Feagans J, Victor D, Moehlen M, Florman SS, Regenstein F, Balart LA, et al. Interstitial pneumonitis in the transplant patient: consider sirolimus-associated pulmonary toxicity. J La State Med Soc. 2009 May-Jun;161(3):166, 8-72.
[69] Perez MJ, Martin RO, Garcia DM, Rey JM, de la Cruz Lombardo J, Rodrigo Lopez JM. Interstitial pneumonitis associated with sirolimus in liver transplantation: a case report. Transplantation proceedings. 2007 Dec;39(10):3498-9.
[70] Howard L, Gopalan D, Griffiths M, Mahadeva R. Sirolimus-induced pulmonary hypersensitivity associated with a CD4 T-cell infiltrate. Chest. 2006 Jun;129(6):1718-21.
[71] Nashan B. Early clinical experience with a novel rapamycin derivative. Therapeutic drug monitoring. 2002 Feb;24(1):53-8.
[72] O'Donnell A, Faivre S, Burris HA, 3rd, Rea D, Papadimitrakopoulou V, Shand N, et al. Phase I pharmacokinetic and pharmacodynamic study of the oral mammalian target of rapamycin inhibitor everolimus in patients with advanced solid tumors. J Clin Oncol. 2008 Apr 1;26(10):1588-95.
[73] Kovarik JM, Hartmann S, Figueiredo J, Rordorf C, Golor G, Lison A, et al. Effect of food on everolimus absorption: quantification in healthy subjects and a confirmatory screening in patients with renal transplants. Pharmacotherapy. 2002 Feb;22(2):154-9.
[74] Kovarik JM, Kahan BD, Kaplan B, Lorber M, Winkler M, Rouilly M, et al. Longitudinal assessment of everolimus in de novo renal transplant recipients over the first post-transplant year: pharmacokinetics, exposure-response relationships, and influence on cyclosporine. Clinical pharmacology and therapeutics. 2001 Jan;69(1):48-56.
[75] Kahan BD, Wong RL, Carter C, Katz SH, Von Fellenberg J, Van Buren CT, et al. A phase I study of a 4-week course of SDZ-RAD (RAD) quiescent cyclosporine-prednisone-treated renal transplant recipients. Transplantation. 1999 Oct 27;68(8):1100-6.
[76] Viklicky O, Zou H, Muller V, Lacha J, Szabo A, Heemann U. SDZ-RAD prevents manifestation of chronic rejection in rat renal allografts. Transplantation. 2000 Feb 27;69(4):497-502.
[77] Eisen HJ, Tuzcu EM, Dorent R, Kobashigawa J, Mancini D, Valantine-von Kaeppler HA, et al. Everolimus for the prevention of allograft rejection and vasculopathy in cardiac-transplant recipients. The New England journal of medicine. 2003 Aug 28;349(9):847-58.

[78] Vitko S, Margreiter R, Weimar W, Dantal J, Viljoen HG, Li Y, et al. Everolimus (Certican) 12-month safety and efficacy versus mycophenolate mofetil in de novo renal transplant recipients. Transplantation. 2004 Nov 27;78(10):1532-40.
[79] Lehmkuhl HB, Arizon J, Vigano M, Almenar L, Gerosa G, Maccherini M, et al. Everolimus with reduced cyclosporine versus MMF with standard cyclosporine in de novo heart transplant recipients. Transplantation. 2009 Jul 15;88(1):115-22.
[80] Pilmore HL, Dittmer ID. Calcineurin inhibitor nephrotoxicity: reduction in dose results in marked improvement in renal function in patients with coexisting chronic allograft nephropathy. Clin Transplant. 2002 Jun;16(3):191-5.
[81] Arora S, Ueland T, Wennerblom B, Sigurdadottir V, Eiskjaer H, Botker HE, et al. Effect of Everolimus Introduction on Cardiac Allograft Vasculopathy-Results of a Randomized, Multicenter Trial. Transplantation. Jun 14.
[82] Griffith BP, Hardesty RL, Deeb GM, Starzl TE, Bahnson HT. Cardiac transplantation with cyclosporin A and prednisone. Annals of surgery. 1982 Sep;196(3):324-9.
[83] Starzl TE, Klintmalm GB, Weil R, 3rd, Porter KA, Iwatsuki S, Schroter GP, et al. Cyclosporin A and steroid therapy in sixty-six cadaver kidney recipients. Surgery, gynecology & obstetrics. 1981 Oct;153(4):486-94.
[84] Starzl TE, Klintmalm GB, Porter KA, Iwatsuki S, Schroter GP. Liver transplantation with use of cyclosporin a and prednisone. The New England journal of medicine. 1981 Jul 30;305(5):266-9.
[85] Andreone PA, Olivari MT, Elick B, Arentzen CE, Sibley RK, Bolman RM, et al. Reduction of infectious complications following heart transplantation with triple-drug immunotherapy. The Journal of heart transplantation. 1986 Jan-Feb;5(1):13-9.
[86] Bolman RM, 3rd, Elick B, Olivari MT, Ring WS, Arentzen CE. Improved immunosuppression for heart transplantation. The Journal of heart transplantation. 1985 May;4(3):315-8.
[87] Hosenpud JD, Bennett LE, Keck BM, Fiol B, Boucek MM, Novick RJ. The Registry of the International Society for Heart and Lung Transplantation: fifteenth official report--1998. J Heart Lung Transplant. 1998 Jul;17(7):656-68.
[88] Hetzer R, Loebe M, Hummel M, Franz N, Schueler S, Friedel N, et al. Heart transplantation in Berlin--1993 update. Clin Transpl. 1993:129-35.
[89] Hershberger RE, Starling RC, Eisen HJ, Bergh CH, Kormos RL, Love RB, et al. Daclizumab to prevent rejection after cardiac transplantation. The New England journal of medicine. 2005 Jun 30;352(26):2705-13.
[90] Baran DA, Zucker MJ, Arroyo LH, Camacho M, Goldschmidt ME, Nicholls SJ, et al. A prospective, randomized trial of single-drug versus dual-drug immunosuppression in heart transplantation: the tacrolimus in combination, tacrolimus alone compared (TICTAC) trial. Circ Heart Fail. Mar 1;4(2):129-37.
[91] Kobashigawa JA. Strategies in immunosuppression after heart transplantation: is less better? Circ Heart Fail. Mar 1;4(2):111-3.
[92] Schweiger M, Wasler A, Prenner G, Tripolt M, Schwarz M, Tscheliessnigg KH. Late acute cardiac allograft rejection: new therapeutic options? Transplantation proceedings. 2005 Dec;37(10):4528-31.

[93] Kobashigawa JA, Stevenson LW, Brownfield ED, Gleeson MP, Moriguchi JD, Kawata N, et al. Corticosteroid weaning late after heart transplantation: relation to HLA-DR mismatching and long-term metabolic benefits. J Heart Lung Transplant. 1995 Sep-Oct;14(5):963-7.

2

Antibody Mediated Rejection of the Cardiac Allograft

Christopher R. Ensor and Christina T. Doligalski
The Johns Hopkins Hospital & Tampa General Hospital, USA

1. Introduction

Antibody mediated rejection (AMR), also known as B-cell mediated rejection or humoral rejection, of the cardiac allograft was first clinically described in the late 1980's (Herskowitz et al., 1987) followed shortly thereafter by pathologic evidence to support a unique rejection process apart from cellular mechanisms (Hammond et al., 1989). This is in contrast to the progression of knowledge regarding cellular rejection, or T-cell mediated rejection, which was readily described in the early 1960's and is the target of most current maintenance immunosuppression agents. Unfortunately, AMR remains poorly understood due, in large measure, to its complicated presentation, pathophysiology, diagnosis, and treatment. The lack of clarity regarding AMR has been compounded by multiple small studies in varying populations with a multitude of treatment modalities and combinations. Additionally, several new agents have been recently utilized or hypothesized to be of utility, with varying success.

Given the complexity of this process, lack of standardization in diagnosis, and multiple proposed treatment options, several professional organizations have endeavored to come to a consensus on the subject of AMR in heart transplant recipients. Most recently in 2011, the International Society for Heart and Lung Transplantation (ISHLT) published their outcomes from a consensus conference regarding AMR in heart transplantation (Kobashigawa et al., 2011) as well as a breakout group working formulation regarding pathologic diagnosis of AMR in heart transplantation (Berry et al., 2011). While these two documents provide some direction for practitioners and transplant providers, many questions remained unanswered and the rapid evolution of novel therapies and strategies for treatment will likely change the field of AMR in the heart transplant population dramatically.

This chapter will look to lay a foundational knowledge of the pathophysiology, epidemiology, and diagnosis of AMR. Additionally, traditional therapies are described and evaluated with a highlight on the controversies surrounding their use; finally, novel and experimental therapies along with their potential impact on prevention and treatment of AMR are described.

2. Definitions

Antibody mediated rejection can be characterized in several different ways. First, it can be qualified based upon the temporal relationship it has to transplantation. Hyperacute AMR is a well known, well described process by which a patient has previously been exposed to some antigen that a donor expresses, and upon transplantation a rapid, immediate antibody response occurs leading to graft dysfunction and most often graft loss within 24 hours. Treatment of hyperacute AMR rarely reverses the process to salvage the graft. Acute AMR occurs sometime after the 24 hour postoperative period, and is generally rapid in onset; treatment strategies may be moderately effective. Chronic or late AMR is a newly recognized, poorly understood process that usually occurs greater than one year following transplantation and is thought to be very slow in progression with poor response to therapy.

Additionally, AMR can be described as either occurring due to pre-sensitization or is the result of *de novo* antibody production. *De novo* AMR occurs when a recipient lacks donor specific antibodies (DSA) and has a negative cross-match at the time of transplant, but subsequently develops AMR at some point after transplantation. Alternatively, if a patient has been previously exposed to antigens that a donor expresses, they are said to be pre-sensitized and typically receive prophylactic or empiric treatment in the peri-operative period. If, however, antibodies reappear at some point in the post-transplant period a renewed AMR may occur.

3. Pathophysiology

The immune system can generally be divided in to two main arms: the T cell, "cellular", arm, and the B cell, "humoral", arm. While these systems are complex and largely integrated, they do originate independently. B cells begin in the bone marrow as progenitor B cells and through activation by encounters with antigens mature through pro B cell, pre B cell, immature, and finally mature B cells. Activated mature B cells are also known as plasma cells and are essentially antibody factories. Antibodies are specific to a single antigen, such as proteins expressed on the surface of a transplanted organ, that are created to attach and signal other parts of the immune system to attack the foreign substance. This immune activation by antibody signaling ultimately damages the allograft. Damage is thought to occur via complement cascade-mediated fixation and activation, which actively damages the foreign material and also acts as a biochemical "amplifier", signaling other parts of the innate and adaptive immune systems such as neutophils, pro-inflammatory molecules and cytokines for example, to relocate to the site of antibody adhesion and attack. One of the more unique aspects of the B cell arm of the immune system is that it retains memory. Once a person has been exposed to an antigen presenting cell (usually from a foreign physiologic source such as an organ or transfusion) and mounts an immune response, a memory B cell is created that, without active intervention, will always exist and will mount a more-rapid response to subsequent antigen presentation from the same source.

These antigens can be portions of viruses, bacteria, or fungus. Human cells also express antigens; the most commonly identified of which are human leukocyte antigens (HLA). While a person does not usually attack itself and therefore tolerates their own HLAs, this is not true for other human tissues that express various antigens and are introduced in to a patient such as in solid organ transplantation.

Subsequently, the risk factors for development of AMR include anything that exposes patients to other human products and therefore creates more potential memory cells to respond to a transplanted organ. These include pregnancies, blood and blood product transfusions, repeat transplantation, and, specific to heart transplantation, the widespread and growing use of extracorporeal and intracorporeal mechanical circulatory support devices such as left ventricular assist systems (LVAS), bi-ventricular assist devices, total artificial hearts, extracorporeal membranous oxygenators (ECMO), or intra-aortic counterpulsators (Reed et al., 2006).

AMR has recently been described as occurring across a spectrum, from completely asymptomatic circulating antibody to clinically overt organ rejection with hemodynamic compromise, graft loss, and decreased survival (Takemoto et al., 2004). Additionally, AMR has been described to contribute significantly to cardiac allograft vasculopathy (CAV), and often occurs in conjunction with acute cellular rejection as so-called mixed rejection (Montgomery et al., 2004).

4. Epidemiology

The true incidence of AMR has been difficult to define given the lack of standardization in diagnosis; however, it is generally accepted that AMR plays a much larger role in overall graft and patient survival than previously appreciated. The reported incidence of *de novo* AMR varies widely based upon the definitions used and at which point on the spectrum a study defines AMR. Epidemiologic studies in centers that perform protocolized endomyocardial biopsies have shown a wide variability in incidence of 3 - 51% (Michaels et al., 2003; Shahzad et al., 2011). Not surprisingly, those institutions that include circulating antibodies without evidence of graft dysfunction had a higher reported incidence of AMR.

Additionally, as the boundaries of transplantation have been expanded in recent years, the number of patients who present for transplantation highly pre-sensitized to other human antigens is on the rise. Based on a survey of the patients who experienced AMR at some point after transplant from 46 heart transplant centers, 35% (114/324) of patients were pre-sensitized prior to transplant, and of those 32% (37/114) were treated to attempt to reduce the amount of circulating antibodies prior to transplantation (Kobashigawa et al., 2011).

5. Diagnosis

Significant effort has been placed on standardizing the diagnosis of AMR of the cardiac allograft within the past 3 - 5 years. These efforts highlight that clinical factors, immunologic criteria, and pathologic criteria all play important roles. In 2004, a general staging of AMR was developed (Table 1), as were criteria for diagnosis of AMR in heart transplant recipients (Table 2). More recently, the ISHLT proposed a preliminary pathologic grading scheme similar to the 2004 guidelines (Table 3) with one major difference: the ISHLT workgroup recognized AMR as a diagnosis that can be made without evidence of circulating antibodies or clinical dysfunction.

5.1 Immunologic screening

Antibody screening tests have been clinically available for many years. These tests determine circulating antibody, but do not address very low level antibodies or antibodies that may be active but not in circulation. Prior to solid-phase antibody (SPA) testing, the presence of antibodies was determined utilizing cell-based assays. The mainstay of testing

	Circulating Antibody	C4d Deposition	Tissue Pathology	Graft Dysfunction
Stage I: Latent Humoral Response	Present			
Stage II: Silent Humoral Rejection	Present	Present		
Stage III: Subclinical Humoral Rejeciton	Present	Present	Present	
Stage IV. Humoral Rejection	Present	Present	Present	Present

Table 1. General AMR staging

Evidence of graft dysfunction	Present
Histologic evidence of tissue injury	*Endothelial swelling or denudation
	*Macrophages in capillaries
	Neutrophils in capillaries
	Interstitial edema, congestion and/or hemorrhage
Immunopathologic evidence for antibody action	Ig G, M, and/or A
	C3d and/or C4d and/or C1q in capillaries
	Fibrin in vessels
Serologic evidence of anti-HLA or other anti-donor antibody at time of biopsy	Present

* required histologic findings

Table 2. 2004 diagnostic criteria of acute AMR in heart transplant recipients

Category	Description	Definition
pAMR 0	Negative for pathologic AMR	Both histologic and immunopathologic studies are negative
pAMR 1 (H+)	Histopathologic AMR alone	Histologic findings present and immunopathologic studies negative
pAMR 1 (I+)	Immunopathologic AMR alone	Histologic findings negative and immunopathologic findings positive
pAMR 2	Pathologic AMR	Both histologic and immunopathologic findings present
pAMR 3	Severe pathologic AMR	Histologic findings of interstitial hemorrhage, capillary fragmentation, mixed inflammatory infiltrates, endothelial cell pyknosis, and/or karyorrhexis and marked edema

Table 3. 2011 ISHLT criteria for pathologic AMR

was complement-dependent cytotoxicity (CDC) assays which involve incubating patient serum with cells of known HLA types, rabbit sera as a source of complement, and finally cell dyes to determine the amount of cell death that has occurred. The HLAs tested cover a very wide spectrum of known HLAs, however not all HLAs are tested. Limitations of this test included its lack of sensitivity and specificity (Berry et al., 2011). Unfortunately, the differences in clinical impact of circulating donor specific antibodies (DSAs), anti-HLA antibodies, or non-HLA antibodies, comparatively, have not been fully elucidated.

5.1.1 Solid Phase Antibody detection

The recent advent of SPA detection has revolutionized immunologic screening. The so-called Luminex® (LABScreen, One Lambda Inc., Canoga Park, CA) single antigen bead (SAB) assay panel provides a comprehensive assessment of individualized IgG and IgM HLA antibodies present in the recipient using a multiplex platform (El-Awar et al., 2005). These beads are coated with fluorescein-tagged antigens, which fluoresce in the presence of the known HLA antibody. The degree of fluorescence, defined in units of mean equivalents of soluble fluorochrome or mean fluorescent intensity, is directly proportional to the circulating amount of the HLA antibody in question. This quantitation is critical when determining which antibodies to exclude from the potential donor pool, and during the depletion process of DSA in the post transplant period.

Despite this improved specificity, the positive predictive value (PPV) of the Luminex assay for AMR remains poor (45%); however, the negative predictive value for AMR is quite good (100%) in a recent analysis (Chin et al., 2011). In an effort to improve the PPV of the Luminex-SAB assay, the Immunogenetics Laboratory at Stanford University spiked an otherwise ordinary Luminex assay sample with purified human Complement-1q (C1q) and ran the sample. The results of the assay revealed a significant decrease in background antibodies, and focused the assay only on those HLA antibodies able to fix C1q. This addition improved the assay's PPV, dramatically, to 100% (Chin et al., 2011). This technique is currently in its infancy, but may result in enhanced utility of the Luminex assay over the decade to come.

5.2 Pathophysiology

Endomyocardial biopsies (EMB) at many centers are routinely performed in addition to those performed for any patient who exhibits signs and symptoms of graft dysfunction. It has been recognized that findings seen on histology are unique from those seen with acute cellular rejection or CAV. Some consensus regarding the findings for AMR was established recently. Pathologic findings are almost exclusively found in the capillary beds; common findings in AMR include endothelial swelling or denudation, deposition of macrophages or neutrophils in capillaries, and interstitial edema, congestion, and potentially hemorrhage in severe cases. Immunopathologic findings include deposition of IgG, M, or A, and positive staining for byproducts of the complement cascade including Complement-3d (C3d), Complement-4d (C4d), or C1q in the capillaries. Sometimes fibrin may also be found in the vessel beds. Table 3 outlines the grading criteria for pathologic AMR staging.

6. Treatment

When discussing treatment options, there are two major divisions for which these therapies have been studied. The first is for the removal of circulating antibodies prior to transplantation, a process known as desensitization; the second is for treatment of AMR, whether it be a reactivation of a previously sensitized patient or *de novo* AMR. Desensitization may be performed to either remove circulating antibody in the weeks to months prior to a transplant in an effort to allow for a larger donor pool in highly sensitized patients, or to mitigate the risk of AMR in the early postoperative period when a patient is known to have mismatched antigens such as is the case with ABO incompatible transplantation or positive cross-matches at the time of transplantation. Treatment may be performed at any point in the spectrum of AMR, from treatment of asymptomatic circulating antibodies to the treatment of clinically significant graft dysfunction caused by antibody-mediated activation of the immune system, with the goals of halting current damage, reverse signs and symptoms of AMR, and long-term to prevent the development of CAV and improve allograft and patient survival. Figure 1 contains a proposed treatment algorithm.

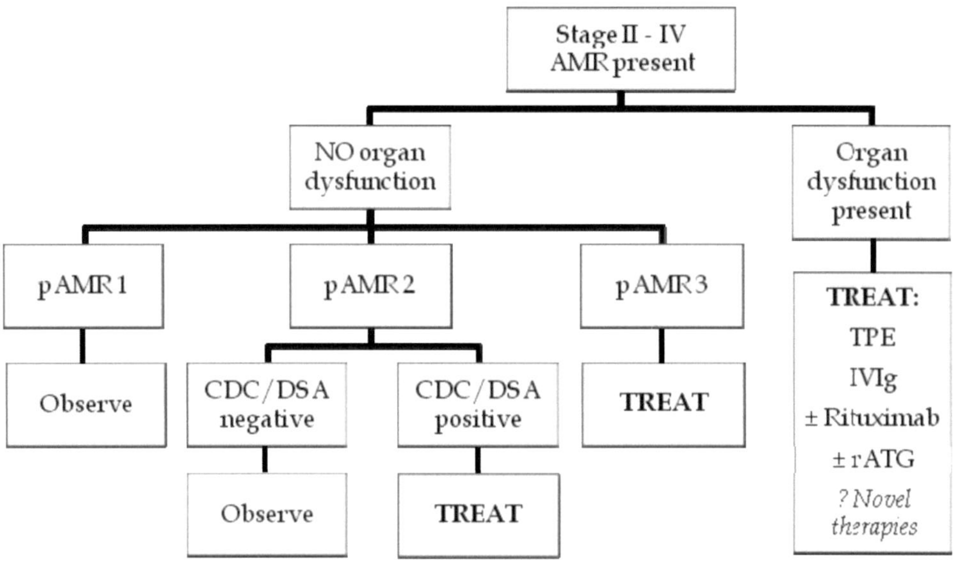

Fig. 1. AMR treatment algorithm. CDC, complement dependent cytotoxicity. DSA, donor specific antibody. IVIg, intravenous immunoglobulins. rATG, rabbit anti-thymocyte globulin. TPE, plasmapheresis.

6.1 Plasmapheresis

Plasmapheresis, or plasma exchange, has been used clinically for a variety of autoimmune conditions since the early 1970's and is generally considered a cornerstone for treatment of AMR. It is a process which physically removes circulating antibodies along with many other circulating proteins; generally 7 – 14 plasmapheresis sessions at varying intervals (from daily to every 3 – 4 days) are required for substantial removal of antibodies. Each session generally lasts 2 – 4 hours. It is an invasive procedure in which a large-bore central venous catheter must be placed and extracorporeal separation of blood occurs via either centrifuge or filtration, antibodies are removed and discarded, and finally blood is returned to the patient.

6.1.1 Plasmapheresis techniques

Three main techniques can be utilized: therapeutic plasma exchange (TPE), double-filtration plasmapheresis (DFPP), and immunoadsorption plasmapheresis (IAPP). Therapeutic plasma exchange involves separation of red blood cells from plasma, complete removal of all plasma, and finally administration of exogenous fresh-frozen plasma or albumin to replace the plasma removed. In many centers, protocols require repletion with both albumin and fresh-frozen plasma on alternating days to replete coagulation factors removed that are not present in exogenous albumin preparations. Double-filtration plasmapheresis separates plasma from red blood cells in the first step, followed by a second filtration of the plasma that separates large molecules from small molecules and sera, and the small molecules and sera are then infused with the endogenous red blood cells. The final technique, immunoadsorption, is theoretically similar to DFPP, but utilizes an immunochemical reaction in the second step to remove only immunoglobulins. TPE and DFPP are older, more established techniques and relatively inexpensive; the immunoadsorbent membrane utilized with IAPP is quite expensive and removes only circulating immunoglobulins, potentially leaving signaling molecules for AMR such as cytokines in circulation. However, an advantage of IAPP is the avoidance of replacement colloids like albumin and fresh-frozen plasma and the adverse effects that are associated with these products; plasma exchange is the predominant method utilized at most US transplant centers.

6.1.2 Data for plasmapheresis in heart transplantation

Plasmapheresis has been utilized significantly in both desensitization protocols as well as in the treatment of AMR in all solid organ transplants as well as heart transplant recipients. Among sensitized patients awaiting transplantation, the preoperative use of plasmapheresis with intravenous immunoglobulins (IVIg) produced similar intermediate term outcomes of rejection and allograft survival compared to non-sensitized patients (Larson et al., 1999; Leech et al., 2006; Pisani et al., 1999). For the treatment of AMR, plasmapheresis has been utilized as part of a multi-treatment modality with success. In 2006, Wang and colleges reported moderate success with 5 days of daily plasma exchange for 12 symptomatic AMR cases in conjunction with methylprednisolone 1gm/day (Wang et al., 2006). In surveying 6 major cardiac transplant centers, all report plasmapheresis as part of their initial management strategy for AMR. Unfortunately, no studies have compared therapy of AMR with or without plasmapheresis, so the actual contribution to good outcomes is impossible to determine at this point, however it is recommended as one of the first line strategies for treatment of AMR (Kobashigawa et al., 2011).

6.1.3 Considerations with plasmapheresis use

One major consideration with use of plasmapheresis is medication removal; medications that are highly protein-bound with low volumes of distribution will be readily removed by TPE or DFPP, and should be administered after the session is complete. In studies evaluating removal of medications in the setting of overdose, those medications with a Vd less than 0.2 L/kg and greater than 80% protein binding were most likely to be substantially removed (Sketris et al., 1984). Case reports have found minimal removal of calcineurin inhibitors, prednisone, or azathioprine (Balogun et al., 2001; Hale et al., 2000; Stigelman et al., 1984); however one case report of plasma exchange following administration of basiliximab found significant removal (Okechukwu et al., 2001). Other agents with likely removal by plasma exchange of concern to transplant recipients include rituximab, (Darabi et al., 2006), vancomycin (Foral & Heineman 2001; Osman & Lew 1997; Sirvent & Borras-Blasco 2006), levothyroxine (Binemelis et al., 1987; Liel et al., 2003), and aminoglycoside antibiotics (Kale-Pradhan et al., 1995; Ouellete et al., 1983; Appelgate et al., 1981). Regardless of likelihood of removal by plasma exchange, every effort should be made to administer critical medications following a session to ensure adequate exposure.

6.2 Total Intravenous Immunoglobulins (IVIg)

Total intravenous immunoglobulins are likely the most often utilized product for desensitization and treatment of AMR across solid organ transplantation including cardiac transplant recipients. IVIg was originally developed in the 1980's as a replacement product for those patients with immune deficiencies, but anti-inflammatory and immunomodulatory effects were quickly understood. The actual mechanisms of immunomodulatory effects of IVIg have been widely postulated, however consensus has not been reached on exactly how IVIg may prevent or halt AMR; rather a "multi-hit" model has been proposed.

6.2.1 Mechanisms of action

Proposed mechanisms specific to the humoral immune system include increased apoptosis of B cells, neutralization of B cell survival signaling molecules, regulation of antibody production, and decreased B cell proliferation (Nimmerjahn & Ravetch 2008; Brandt & Gershwin 2006; Jordan & Toyoda 2009; Durandy et al., 2009). A multitude of mechanisms that affect other aspects of the immune system including T cells, neutrophils, NK cells, and so forth have been proposed as well. Dose-dependent effects have also been proposed, with low-doses (500 mg/kg) IVIg reported to have more pro-inflammatory effects whereas high-doses (1 – 2 gm/kg) exhibit anti-inflammatory and more immunoregulatory effects.

6.2.2 Data for IVIg in heart transplantation

While IVIg is one of the most common agents used in AMR of the cardiac allograft, data are surprisingly limited for its use. Four main studies have evaluated the utility of IVIg for desensitization prior to cardiac transplantation. Similar to the data seen with other therapy modalities, IVIg has been used in combination with either plasmapheresis, rituximab, or high dose corticosteroids. No studies have shown that IVIg alone can reduce antibody burden pre-transplant, and outcomes following successful transplant are conflicting (Shehata et al., 2010; Nussinovitch & Shoenfeld 2008; Pisani et al., 1999; John et al., 1999). In the treatment of AMR, data are more robust; although again no studies have evaluated the utility of IVIg alone.

6.2.3 Considerations with IVIg Use

One unique consideration for the use of IVIg is product selection. Currently, seven FDA approved products are available for use. The major considerations for product selection are stabilizing agents/sugar contents, the IgA content, anti-A and anti-B isohemagglutinin concentrations, and availability of the product. One of the known adverse effects of high-dose IVIg therapy is acute kidney injury (AKI). The likely contributors to AKI are sheer protein load, osmolarity, and the excipient content of the product. Higher doses and therefore higher protein loads are associated with increased rates of adverse effects, as are products with sucrose as an excipient and those with high osmolarities. Efforts to decrease these effects include preparations that are liquid products with iso-osmolarity; unfortunately, the techniques utilized to achieve a more tolerable product have increased the titers of anti-isohemagluttinins. These products have therefore been associated with increased rates of clinically significant hemolysis. Clinical monitoring of patients with A, B, or AB blood types with prolonged duration or high doses of IVIg therapy is recommended (Jordan et al., 2011). Additionally, the IgA concentration varies across the available products. IgA depleted products must be used for patients with IgA deficiencies or antibodies to IgA, as IgA rich products may increase the risk of serious adverse reactions such as anaphylaxis. Finally, since IVIg is a pooled human product, it is limited by availability of donors and product demand. Subsequently, intermittent product shortage has been commonplace.

Cytomegalovirus hyperimmune globulin (CMVIg, Cytogam), has a unique historical perspective in solid organ transplantation. While CMVIg has been studied as specific prophlyaxis for cytomegalovirus (CMV) disease, at one point in time, supply of IVIg was greatly limited. During this IVIg shortage, centers utilized the one IVIg product that was available: CMVIg. Subsequently, many centers established efficacy for CMVIg in desensitization and the treatment of AMR, and continue to use this specific product, despite no known or theoretical advantages over total IVIg, purely for immunoregulatory effects.

6.3 Total Lymphoid Irradiation

Total lymphoid irradiation (TLI) is low dose, targeted radiotherapy directed at major concentrations of lymph nodes across the body as well as the spleen. This traditionally has involved radiation exposure to 3 major areas across the body: the first being the chest above the diaphragm and below the base of the skull, a peri-aortic and splenic field, and finally a pelvic field to encompass all pelvic and inguinal lymph nodes. By irradiating these areas, theoretically a long-term decrease in antibody production would occur and mitigate the contribution of the B-cell immune system to rejection and any subsequent rejection episodes (Salter et al., 1995).

TLI has been utilized in the treatment of rejection among solid organ transplant recipients for more than 20 years. The majority of data supporting TLI in the treatment of cardiac AMR comes from a single center, which reported TLI therapy for recurrent rejection or rejection with hemodynamic compromise in 73 patients between 1990 and 1996. TLI was delivered as 80 cGy twice weekly for a total of 5 weeks, and was associated with a significant reduction in risk of rejection. This benefit was seen for approximately 4 years. No changes in long-term outcomes such as CAV or survival were seen. Unfortunately, myelodysplasia (MDS) or acute myelogenous leukemia (AML) did develop in 7 patients. This reported risk of leukemias has significantly limited the utility of TLI, and has lead to consensus recommendations to avoid its use in treatment of AMR (Kobashigawa et al., 2011).

6.4 Photopheresis

Extracoroporeal photopheresis (ECP) is a procedure similar to plasmapheresis where approximately 700mL of blood is removed and separated. The plasma is then incubated with a photosensitizing agent, 8-methoxypsoralen, under UV-A radiation. This process covalently binds the photosensitizing agent to DNA and cell surface. These irradiated lymphocytes, monocytes, and dendritic cells decrease down-stream signaling for immune activation. Although the exact mechanisms are unknown, it is not believed that photopheresis has a majority of its benefit on B cells, but rather T cells; specifically T regulatory cells are affected. Each session is performed for approximately 1 - 3 hours, and sessions vary from daily to weekly.

6.4.1 Data for photopheresis in heart transplantation

ECP gained popularity in the heart transplant population for prevention of rejection when results from a multi-center randomized control trial evaluating standard immunosuppression with or without ECP found a 2 fold decrease in overall incidence of acute rejection. In this study, ECP was performed 2 days in a row every week for 4 weeks, then every 2 weeks for 2 months, and finally every month for 3 months (Barr et al., 1998). Unfortunately, there was no decrease in time to rejection or incidence of rejection with hemodynamic compromise. No studies to date have been performed to specifically evaluate the role of ECP in prophylaxis or treatment of AMR, although the Barr study did demonstrate a significant reduction in HLA antibody levels.

6.4.2 Considerations with photopheresis use

One consideration to be taken regarding photopheresis is the requirement for a central venous catheter; however, it is reported to be better tolerated than plasmapheresis, has minimal side effects, and has been shown to be safe in case reports of heart transplant recipients up to 3 years (Marques & Schwartz 2011). Reported adverse effects include malaise, low-grade fever, and gastrointestinal upset. Risks associated with invasive central lines, such as infection and thrombosis, are present as well.

6.5 Cyclophosphamide

Cyclophosphamide is an alkylating nitrogen mustard chemotherapeutic agent that was approved by the FDA in 1959 and has been used to treat a variety of neoplastic and autoimmune conditions. Its cytotoxic effects arise from intra- and interstrand DNA cross-linking, leading to DNA inactivation and cell death; immunosuppression arises from selective suppression of B-lymphocyte activity as well as a general lymphopenia of both B cells and T cells. Theoretically, cyclophosphamide provides the advantage of avoidance of rebound B cell proliferation with more short-term strategies like plasmapheresis and IVIg that do not alter B cell production.

6.5.1 Data for cyclophosphamide use in heart transplantation

Several small case series have reported success with the use of cyclophosphamide and IVIg for desensitization prior to cardiac transplantation. The first reported a PRA decrease from 64% to 14% with the combination of IVIg and cyclophosphamide, leading to successful transplantation (De Marco et al., 1997). More recently, Itescu and colleagues reported their experience with 16 sensitized LVAS patients awaiting cardiac transplantation, who received monthly treatment with cyclophosphamide 0.5 - 1 g/m2; all 23 patients were successfully transplanted. No differences in adverse events compared to other sensitized patients occurred in this single center experience (Itescu et al., 2002).

6.5.2 Considerations with cyclophosphamide use

The clinical utility of cyclophosphamide, however, has been limited by the potential adverse effect profile and the increased utilization of B cell specific monoclonal antibodies. Primary toxicities associated with cyclophosphamide use include hematologic toxicities, hemorrhagic cystitis, and infertility/teratogenicity. Additionally, there is a risk of secondary malignancies such as leukemia, lymphoma, and skin cancers.

6.6 Anti-Thymocyte Globulin (ATG and rATG)

Anti-thymocyte globulins are polyclonal antibody products derived from either equine (ATG or Atgam®) or leporine (rATG or Thymoglobulin®) sources. Horses or rabbits are inoculated with human lymphocytes; serum is then removed from the animals and the antibodies against human CD3-bearing T cells are collected and purified. These products have been used generously throughout solid organ transplantation as both induction agents at the time of transplant as well as agents for the treatment of rejection, with a shift in clinical practice to almost exclusive use of the rabbit preparation based on studies showing better tolerability and potentially improved outcomes.

6.6.1 Data for Anti-Thymocyte Globulin in heart transplantation

While ATG has been utilized extensively in heart transplant recipients, no studies have evaluated their use in AMR; rather decreased overall rejection rates have been reported (Renlund et al., 1989; Ladowski et al., 1993; Macdonald et al., 1993; Schnetzler et al., 2002; De Santo et al., 2004). In both induction and rejection protocols, daily infusions are given for as little as 3 to at most 14 days. Additionally, no desensitization protocols have reported to utilize ATG. Given the lack of data, however, there is a theoretical benefit for the use of these polyclonal antibodies in the treatment of AMR or mixed ACR/AMR. While the majority of antibodies derived are against T-cells, many other cells are potentially affected, including B-cells, HLA heavy chains, plasma cells, platelets, white blood cells, red blood cells, and so on. In fact, the dose-limiting side effects are typically thrombocytopenia and leucopenia.

6.6.2 Considerations with Anti-Thymocyte Globulin use

In addition to pancytopenia, both products are associated with significant infusion reactions, cytokine release syndrome, and rarely anaphylactic reactions. These infusion reactions are significantly more pronounced in patients that have repeated previous exposure to either source animal and depending on the patient's history may warrant avoidance of a particular product. Pre-medication prior to the infusion with steroids, acetaminophen, and diphenhydramine are recommended. More serious adverse effects include serum sickness, which presents as a delayed reaction with flu-like symptoms, lymphadenopathy, blurred vision, and rash. At the cellular level, increased levels of IgG, IgM, IgE, and acute phase reactants are seen with serum sickness reactions. The effects on humoral activation of serum sickness are as yet unknown.

6.7 Rituximab

Rituximab is a chimeric humanized high-affinity monoclonal antibody targeted against the CD-20 receptor, which is borne by both B-cell progenitors and mature B-lymphocytes. B-cell depletion with rituximab occurs via three mechanisms: complement-dependent cytotoxicity, antibody-dependent cytotoxicity, and induction of apoptosis (Smith, 2003). Problematically, rituximab is only efficacious against circulating B-cells and progenitors and does not penetrate the spleen; thus, should be most efficacious against *de novo* antibodies which have been quickly recognized and intervened upon. In contrast, long-standing antibodies, such as those present in pre-sensitized candidates, should be relatively resistant to rituximab as the plasma cell from which they are generated is no longer circulating in the central compartment.

6.7.1 Data for rituximab in heart transplantation

Rituximab has been used across the spectrum of solid organ transplant recipients both for desensitization and AMR, albeit with minimal quality evidence of efficacy. The data describing rituximab use in cardiac transplantation is case report and case series in nature. Problematically, such case reports describe the addition of rituximab to traditional therapies such as TPE, IVIg, cyclophosphamide, and ATG complicating the evaluation of the efficacy of rituximab alone. Regimens used are also heterogeneous, ranging from 375 mg/m^2 to 1 gram fixed dose for 1 to 4 doses once weekly to twice monthly (Kcazmarek et al., 2007). Given this, it is nearly impossible to quantitate the potential benefit or role of rituximab for AMR in the cardiac allograft. Rigorous evaluation in a systematic fashion of rituximab therapy is desperately needed.

6.7.2 Considerations with rituximab use

Rituximab is generally well tolerated; however, some severe adverse effects have been reported. Leucopenia is relatively common after administration owing in large measure to suppression of B-lymphocyte differentiation. Hemodynamic effects, particularly transient hypotension, have been reported. Anaphylaxis is possible, but incredibly rare. Initially, small rituximab test-doses were required to evaluate anaphylaxis risk; however, these have been relegated due to poor positive predictive value. Since rituximab depletes CD-20 bearing B-cell progenitors, it may be associated with an increased risk of recurrent infections; particularly those of a viral nature that rely on innate memory B-cells for protection such as CMV. The data regarding infectious risk in transplant recipients is qualitatively poor. In a case series of 8 cardiac transplant recipients, 3 patients developed infections (Garrett et al., 2005).

7. Novel and experimental therapies

Recently, alternatives to the previously discussed and more traditional therapies have emerged. These agents target plasma cells both in circulation and in the spleen, B-cell activating factors (BAFF), and the complement cascade. It should be noted that, at present, data supporting the use of these agents in cardiac transplantation is minimal. However, as is the case with many of the traditional therapies, these agents have both been used or are being actively studied in highly sensitized renal transplant recipients (RTR).

7.1 Plasma cell targeted agents

Bortezomib, a 26S proteasomal inhibitor, results in the selective apoptosis of highly active plasma cells both in circulation and in the spleen. The proteasome is responsible for proteolysis of misfolded, damaged, or unneeded proteins within the cell; the inhibition of which leads to cell-cycle arrest and apoptosis (Everly et al., 2008). Only one case report has been published that describes the efficacy of bortezomib for refractory AMR in a cardiac transplant recipient (Eckman et al., 2009). Likewise, only one case series of 7 patients has been reported that describes the successful use of bortezomib for desensitization in candidates refractory to traditional therapies (Patel et al., 2010). The use of bortezomib is likely to expand in cardiac transplantation; particularly as longer-term safety data emerges.

Belimumab is targeted at the BAFF B-lymphocyte stimulator (BLyS) and proliferation-inducing ligand (APRIL). Targeting these tumor necrosis factor-family ligands ultimately results in the apoptosis of mature B-lymphocytes via suppression of BLyS and APRIL-mediated antiapopototic effects during B-cell differentiation and maturation (Bossen & Schneider, 2006). This agent has shown promise in the treatment of systemic lupus erythematosis and is being actively trialed for desensitization in renal transplant candidates.

7.2 Complement cascade targeted agents

Eculizumab, a humaninzed anti-C5 monoclonal antibody, depresses the formation of the membrane attack complex (C5b9) in response to circulating DSA. There are no such reports describing the use of this agent in cardiac transplant recipients; however, 5 anecdotal cases are known to us. In all cases, eculizumab was paired either with traditional means of antibody depletion (TPE and IVIg), bortezomib, or both. A larger experience is known in renal transplantation. Eculizumab was given as prophylaxis of AMR in 10 highly sensitized RTR who received pre-transplant desensitization with TPE and IVIg. Half of the patients developed high DSA titers post-transplant, but no incidences of AMR were recorded in 12 months of follow-up (Stegall, M., et al. 2009). Additionally, eculizumab was given as sole treatment to 16 highly sensitized RTR, and compared to a similarly sensitized cohort of patients who did not receive therapy. The incidence of AMR in the first post-transplant month was substantially less in the eculizumab patients (6.25% vs. 40%); however, 6 patients developed chronic AMR (Cornell et al., 2010). This suggests that eculizumab may be best-utilized when paired with antibody-depletion measures, such as TPE. It should be noted that combining eculizumab with rituximab will render rituximab ineffective as its predominant pro-apoptotic mechanism is complement-mediated.

Cinryze, human C1-esterase inhibitor, is collected from human donors in whole blood, purified via pasteurization and nanofiltration, and is currently approved for hereditary angioedema. The potential role of supraphysiologic concentrations of human C1-esterase inhibitor in the downregulation of the complement cascade notwithstanding, no reports currently exist that describe the role of Cinryze in transplant recipients. However, Cinryze is being actively studied in renal transplantation and may provide an alternative for C5b9 inhibition.

8. Conclusions

Antibody-mediated rejection is a poorly characterized, understood, and studied disease process in solid organ transplantation today. There are active efforts across all organ systems to better-define the pathogenesis of DSA in the development of AMR, the long-term consequences of its development, and the best methodology to screen and manage patients who are pre-sensitized. Relative to AMR in the heart transplant community, until the newly derived definition of AMR is uniformly adopted and utilized, it is unlikely that quality retrospective research will be completed on a large scale. However, there are ongoing efforts at high-volume centers to study the novel and experimental therapies in an effort to enhance transplantability of highly-sensitized candidates and manage AMR when it subsequently develops. Traditional measures, such as TPE and IVIg, remain the cornerstone of AMR therapy. TLI, photophoresis, and cyclophosphamide have fallen out of favor due to adverse effects or lack of efficacy. The role of rituximab is unclear as it has never been subjected to rigorous clinical evaluation and has mechanistic disadvantages relative to its novel alternative, bortezomib. Finally, the horizon is bright for the use of complement-antagonists to reshape how we manage pre-sensitized patients in an effort to enhance their candidacy for transplantation.

9. References

Appelgate, R., Schwartz, D., & Bennett, W. (1981). Removal of tobramycin during plasma exchange therapy. *Annals of Internal Medicine,* Vol. 94, No. 6 (June 1981), pp. 820-1, ISSN 0003-4819

Balogun, R., Sahadevan, M., Sevigney, J., et al. (2001). Impact of therapeutic plasma exchange on cyclosporine kinetics during membrane-based lipid apheresis. *American Journal of Kidney Diseases,* Vol. 37, No. 6, (June 2001), pp. 1286-9, ISSN 1138-2700

Barr, M., Meiser, B., Eisen H., et al. (1998). Photopheresis for the prevention of rejection in cardiac transplantation. *New England Journal of Medicine,* Vol. 339, No. 24, (December 1998), pp. 1744-51, ISSN 0028-4793

Berry, G., Angelini, A., Burke M., et al. (2011). The ISHLT working formulation for pathologic diagnosis of antibody-mediated rejection in heart transplantation: Evolution and current status (2005–2011). *The Journal of Heart and Lung Transplantation,* Vol. 30, No. 6, (June 2011), pp. 601-611, ISSN 2155-5100

Binimelis, J., Bassas, L., Marruecos, L., et al. (1987). Massive thyroxine intoxication: evaluation of plasma extraction. *Intensive Care Medicine,* Vol. 13, No. 1, pp. 33-8, ISSN 355-8934

Bossen, C., & Schneider, P. (2006). BAFF, APRIL and their receptors: Structure, function and signaling. *Seminars in Immunology* Vol. 18, No. 5, (October 2006), pp. 263-75, ISSN 1691-4324

Brandt, D., & Gershwin, M. (2006). Common variable immune deficiency and autoimmunity. *Autoimmunity Reviews,* Vol. 5, No. 7 (August 2006), pp. 465-70, ISSN 1692-0573

Chin, C., Chen, G., Sequeria, F., et al. (2011). Clinical usefulness of a novel C1q assay to detect immunoglobulin G antibodies capable of fixing complement in sensitized pediatric heart transplant patients. *Journal of Heart and Lung Transplantation* Vol. 30, No. 2, (February 2011), pp. 158-63, ISSN 2095-1058

Cornell, L., Gloor, J., Nasr S., et al. (2010). Chronic humoral rejection despite C5 inhibition after positive-crossmatch kidney transplantation. *American Journal of Transplantation* Vol. 10, pp.A125

Darabi, K., & Berg, A. (2006). Rituximab can be combined with daily plasma exchange to achieve effective B-cell depletion and clinical improvement in acute autoimmune TTP. *American Journal of Clinical Pathology* Vol. 125, No. 4 (April 2006), pp. 592-7, ISSN 1662-7268

De Marco, T., Damon, L., Colombe, B., et al. (1997). Successful immunomodulation with intravenous gamma globulin and cyclophosphamide in an alloimmunized heart transplant recipient. *Journal of Heart and Lung Transplantation* Vol. 16, No. 3 (March 1997), pp. 360-5, ISSN 908-7880

De Santo, L., Della Corte, A., Romano, G., et al. (2004). Midterm results of a prospective randomized comparison of two different rabbit-antithymocyte globulin induction therapies after heart transplantation. *Transplantation Proceedings* Vol. 36, No. 3 (April 2004), pp. 631-7, ISSN 1511-0616

Durandy, A., Kaveri, S., Kuijpers, T., et al. (2009). Intravenous immunoglobulins--understanding properties and mechanisms. *Clinical and Experimental Immunology* Vol. 158, Suppl 1 (December 2009), pp. 2-13, ISSN 1988-3419

Eckman, P., Thorsgard, M., Maurer, D., et al. (2009). Bortezomib for refractory antibody-mediated cardiac allograft rejection. *Clinical Transplants* (2009), pp. 475-8, ISSN 2052-4318

El-Awar, N., Lee, J., Terasaki, P., et al. (2005). HLA antibody identification with single antigen beads compared to conventional methods. *Human Immunology* Vol. 66, No. 9 (September 2005), pp. 989-97, ISSN 1636-0839

Everly, J., Walsh, R., Alloway, R., et al. (2009). Proteasome inhibition for antibody-mediated rejection. *Current Opinion in Organ Transplantation* Vol. 14, No. 6 (December 2009), pp. 662-6, ISSN 1966-7989

Foral, M., & Heineman, S. (2001). Vancomycin removal during a plasma exchange transfusion. *Annals of Pharmacotherapy* Vol. 35, No. 11 (November 2001), pp. 1400-2, ISSN 1172-4092

Garrett, H., Duvall-Seaman, D., Helsley, B., et al. (2005). Treatment of vascular rejection with rituximab in cardiac transplantation. *Journal of Heart and Lung Transplantation* Vol. 24, No. 9 (September 2005), pp. 628-30, ISSN 1614-3254

Hale, G., Reece, D., Munn R., et al. (2000). Blood tacrolimus concentrations in bone marrow transplant patients undergoing plasmapheresis. *Bone Marrow Transplantation* Vol. 25, No. 4 (February 2000), pp. 449-51, ISSN 1072-3590

Hammond, E., Yowell, R., Nunoda, S., et al. (1989). Vascular (humoral) rejection in heart transplantation (pathologic observations and clinical implications). *Journal of Heart Transplantation* Vol. 8, No. 6 (November - December 1989), pp. 430-43, ISSN 269-3662

Herskowitz, A, Soule, L.M., Ueda, K., et al. (1987). Arteriolar vasculitis on endomyocardial biopsy: A histologic predictor of poor outcome in cyclosporine-treated heart transplant recipients. *Journal of Heart Transplantation* Vol. 6, No. 3 (May - June 1987), pp. 127-36, ISSN 330-9214

Itescu, S., Burke, S., Lietz, K., et al. (2002). Intravenous pulse administration of cyclophosphamide is an effective and safe treatment for sensitized cardiac allograft recipients. *Circulation* Vol. 105, No. 10 (March 2002), pp. 1214-9, ISSN 1188-9016

Jordan, S., Toyoda, M., Kahwaji, J., et al. (2011). Clinical aspects of intravenous immunoglobulin use in solid organ transplant recipients. *American Journal of Transplantation* Vol. 11, No. 2 (February 2011), pp. 196-202, ISSN 2121-9579

Jordan, S., Toyoda, M., & Vo, A. (2009). Intravenous immunoglobulin a natural regulator of immunity and inflammation. *Transplantation* Vol. 88, No. 1 (July 2009), pp. 1-6, ISSN 1958-4672

Kaczmarek, I., Deutsch, M.A., Sadoni, S., et al. (2007). Successful management of antibody-mediated cardiac allograft rejection with combined immunoadsorption and Anti-CD20 monoclonal antibody treatment: Case report and literature review. *Journal of Heart and Lung Transplantation* Vol. 26, No. 5 (May 2007), pp. 511-5, ISSN 1744-9422

Kale-Pradhan, P., Dehoorne-Smith, M., Jawowrski, D., et al. (1995). Evaluation of plasmapheresis on the removal of tobramycin. *Pharmacotherapy* Vol. 15, No. 5 (September - October 1995), pp. 673-6, ISSN 857-0442

Kobashigawa J, Crespo-Leiro M., Ensminger S., et al. (2011). Report from a consensus conference on antibody-mediated rejection in heart transplantation. *Journal of Heart and Lung Transplantation*, Vol. 30, No. 3 (March 2011), pp. 252-69, ISSN 2130-0295

Ladowski, J., Dillon, T., Schatzlein, M., et al. (1993). Prophylaxis of heart transplant rejection with either antithymocyte globulin-, Minnesota antilymphocyte globulin-, or an OKT3-based protocol. *Journal of Cardiovascular Surgery* (Torino) Vol. 34, No. 2 (April 1993), pp. 135-40, ISSN 832-0247

Larson, D., Elkund, D., Arabia, F., et al. (1999). Plasmapheresis during cardiopulmonary bypass: a proposed treatment for presensitized cardiac transplantation patients. *Journal of Extra Corporeal Technology* Vol. 31, No. 4 (December 1999), pp. 177-83, ISSN 1091-5474

Leech, S., Lopez-Cepero, M., LeFor, W., et al. (2006). Management of the sensitized cardiac recipient: the use of plasmapheresis and intravenous immunoglobulin. *Clinical Transplantation* Vol. 20, No. 4 (July - August 2006), pp. 476-84, ISSN 1684-2525

Liel, Y. & Weksler, N. (2003). Plasmapheresis rapidly eliminates thyroid hormones from the circulation, but does not affect the speed of TSH recovery following prolonged suppression. *Hormone Research* Vol. 60, No. 5 pp. 252-4, ISSN 1461-4231

Macdonald, P., Mundy, J., Keogh, A.M., et al. (1993). A prospective randomized study of prophylactic OKT3 versus equine antithymocyte globulin after heart transplantation--increased morbidity with OKT3. *Transplantation* Vol. 55, No. 1 (January 1993), pp. 110-6, ISSN 838-0508

Marques, M. & Schwartz, J. (2011). Update on extracorporeal photopheresis in heart and lung transplantation. *Journal of Clinical Apheresis* Vol. 26, No. 3 pp. 146-51, ISSN 2164-7952

Michaels, P., Fishbein, M., & Colvin, R. (2003). Humoral rejection of human organ transplants. *Springer Semininars in Immunopathology* Vol. 25, No. 2 (September 2003), pp. 119-40, ISSN 1295-5463

Montgomery, R., Hardy, M., Jordan S., et al. (2004). Consensus opinion from the antibody working group on the diagnosis, reporting, and risk assessment for antibody-mediated rejection and desensitization protocols. *Transplantation* Vol. 78, No. 2 (July 2004), pp. 181-5, ISSN 1528-0674

Nimmerjahn, F. & Ravetch, J. (2008). Anti-inflammatory actions of intravenous immunoglobulin. *Annual Review of Immunology* Vol. 26, pp. 513-33, ISSN 1837-0923

Nussinovitch, U. & Shoenfeld, Y. (2008). Intravenous immunoglobulin - indications and mechanisms in cardiovascular diseases. *Autoimmunity Reviews* Vol. 7, No. 6, pp. 445-52, ISSN 1855-8360

Okechukwu, C., Meier-Kriesche, H., Armstrong, D., et al. (2001). Removal of basiliximab by plasmapheresis. *American Journal of Kidney Diseases* Vol. 37, No. 1 (January 2001), pp. E11, ISSN 1113-6200

Osman, B. & Lew, S. (1997). Vancomycin removal by plasmapheresis. *Pharmacology and Toxicology* Vol. 81, No. 5 (November 1997), pp. 245-6, ISSN 939-6092

Ouellette, S., Visconti, J., & Kennedy, M. (1983). A pharmacokinetic evaluation of the effect of plasma exchange on tobramycin disposition. *Clinical and Experimental Dialysis and Apheresis* Vol. 7, No. 3, pp. 225-33, ISSN 667-1353

Patel, J., Kittleson, M., Reed, E., et al. (2010). The effectiveness of a standardized desensitization protocol in reducing calculated panel reactive antibodies (cPRA) in sensitized heart transplant candidates: does it make sense to desensitize? *Journal of Heart and Lung Transplantation* Vol. 29, pp. S103-4

Pisani, B., Mullen, G., Malinowska, K., et al. (1999). Plasmapheresis with intravenous immunoglobulin G is effective in patients with elevated panel reactive antibody prior to cardiac transplantation. *Journal of Heart and Lung Transplantation* Vol. 18, No. 7, (July 1999), pp. 701-6, ISSN 1045-2347

Reed, E., Demetris, A., Hammond, E., et al. (2006). Acute antibody-mediated rejection of cardiac transplants. *Journal of Heart and Lung Transplantation* Vol. 25, No. 2 (February 2006), pp.153-9, ISSN 1644-6213

Renlund, D., O'Connell, J., & Bristow, M. (1989). Early rejection prophylaxis in heart transplantation: is cytolytic therapy necessary? *Journal of Heart Transplantation* Vol. 8, No. 3 (May - June 1989), pp. 191-3, ISSN 266-1767

Salter, S., Salter, M., Kirklin, J., et al. (1995). Total lymphoid irradiation in the treatment of early or recurrent heart transplant rejection. *International Journal of Radiation Oncoogy,l Biology, and Physics* Vol. 33, No. 1 (August 1995), pp. 83-8, ISSN 764-2435

Schnetzler, B., Leger, P., Volp, A., et al. (2002). A prospective randomized controlled study on the efficacy and tolerance of two antilymphocytic globulins in the prevention of rejection in first-heart transplant recipients. *Transplantation International* Vol. 15, No. 6 (June 2002), pp. 317-25, ISSN 1207-2903

Shahzad, K., Aziz, Q., Leva J., et al. (2011). New-onset graft dysfunction after heart transplantation--incidence and mechanism-related outcomes. *Journal of Heart and Lung Transplantation* Vol. 30, No. 2 (February 2011), pp. 194-203, ISSN 2095-2209

Shehata, N., Palda, V., Meyer, R., et al. (2010). The use of immunoglobulin therapy for patients undergoing solid organ transplantation: an evidence-based practice guideline. *Transfusion Medicine Reviews* Vol. 24, Suppl. 1 (January 2010), pp. S7-S27, ISSN 1996-2580

Sirvent, A., Borras-Blasco, J., Enriquez, R., et al. (2006). Extracorporeal removal of vancomycin by plasmapheresis. *Annals of Pharmacotherapy* Vol. 40, No. 12 (December 2006), pp. 2279-80, ISSN 1713-2808

Smith, M. (2003). Rituximab (monoclonal anti-CD20 antibody): mechanisms of action and resistance. *Oncogene* Vol. 22, No. 47 (October 2003), pp. 7359-68, ISSN 1457-6843

Stegall, M., Diwan. T., Burns, J., et al. (2009). Prevention of acute humoral rejection with C5 inhibition. *American Journal of Transplantation* Vol. 9, pp. A178

Stigelman, W. Jr., Henry, D., Talbert, R., et al. (1984). Removal of prednisone and prednisolone by plasma exchange. *Clinical Pharmacy* Vol. 3, No. 4 (July – August 1984), pp. 402-7, ISSN 646-7876

Takemoto, S. K., Zeevi, A., Feng, S., et al. (2004). National conference to assess antibody-mediated rejection in solid organ transplantation. *American Journal of Transplantation* Vol. 4, No. 7 (July 2004), pp. 1033-41, ISSN 1519-6059

Wang, S. S., Chou, N., Ko, W., et al. (2006). Effect of plasmapheresis for acute humoral rejection after heart transplantation. *Transplantation Proceedings* Vol. 38, No. 10 (December 2006), pp. 3692-4, ISSN 1717-5369

3

Nutritional Intervention in Heart Transplant Recipients – Dietary Recommendations

Paloma Posada-Moreno et al.*
Universidad Complutense de Madrid, Spain

1. Introduction

Timely nutrition assessment and intervention in organ transplant recipients may improve outcomes surrounding transplantation. Because nutritional status is a potentially modifiable risk factor, the development of strategies designed to optimize nutritional status decreases the short-term risks in the post transplant period (Russo et al., 2010).

Despite many advances in surgical techniques, diagnostic approaches and immunosuppressive strategies, survival after heart transplantation is limited by the development of cardiac allograft vasculopathy (CAV) which is the most important cause of death late after transplantation (Hosenpud et al., 1998; Pethig et al., 1997) and by the adverse effects of immunosuppression.

Primary prevention of CAV in heart transplant (HT) recipients should include strict control of cardiovascular risk factors (hypertension, diabetes, hyperlipidemia, smoking and obesity), as well as strategies for the prevention of cytomegalovirus (CMV) infection (Costanzo et al., 2010). The sum of various risk factors has a negative impact on survival (Almenar et al., 2005). In addition, malnutrition increases the risk of infection post transplant and may reduce survival (Hasse, 2001).

It has been referenced that improper dietary habits, low physical activity and the side effects of immunosuppressive therapy might explain the weight gain, the altered lipid pattern and an increase in insulin resistance after transplant (Evangelista et al., 2005; Flattery et al., 2006; Uddén et al., 2003). The metabolic picture after transplantation is also worsened by the immunosuppressive drugs (Anker et al., 1997; Kemna et al., 1994). Therefore, the development of strategies to reduce post transplant body weight and to improve insulin resistance is important (Sénéchal, 2005).

Immunosuppressive agents, such as prednisone, cyclosporine, mycophenylate mofetil and sirolimus, are associated with hyperlipidemia (Bilchick, 2004). The glucocorticoids play a major role in the development of post transplant osteoporosis (Epstein & Shane, 1996; Epstein et al., 1995; Glendenning et al., 1999; Reid et al., 1988; Rodino & Shane, 1998; Shane, 2000; Stempfle et al., 1999) and it is known that side effects of glucocorticoids, such as on

* Ismael Ortuño-Soriano, Ignacio Zaragoza-García, Mª Dolores Rodríguez-Martínez, José Luis Pacheco-del-Cerro, Carmen Martínez-Rincón and Antonio Luis Villarino-Marín

weight gain and the increase of appetite (Kahn & Flier, 2000; Uddén et al., 2003), may induce insulin resistance and diabetes mellitus.

Osteoporosis is a leading cause of morbidity; the most rapid bone loss occurs during the first three months and in the first two years after cardiac transplantation (Hasse, 2001; Henderson et al., 1995).

In addition, statins are usually required in transplant recipients to achieve low LDL cholesterol levels. High concentrations of these drugs, particularly in combination with cyclosporine, may increase the risk of side effects (Vorlat et al., 2003).

Recommendations for specific levels of nutrients should be made after the following factors are considered: nutritional status, body weight, age, gender, metabolic state, stage and type of organ failure, presence of infection, malabsorption or induced losses, goals and comorbid conditions (Hasse, 2001).

The effectiveness of nutritional education should consider a number of psychological variables, including social, cultural and ethnicity factors. These variables are present when HT recipients return to their usual context. Although not a priority for the survival of the person, they are important to the goal of the nutritional action.

Finally, HT recipients should be provided with a multidisciplinary team, including surgeons, cardiologist, nurses, psychologists and dieticians, among many others including ancillary services, such as home care nursing, cardiac rehabilitation, psychologic support, nutritional planning or patient support groups that can be used as resources in the follow-up of HT recipients (Costanzo et al., 2010).

2. Nutritional assessment

A comprehensive nutritional assessment of transplant recipients should include a variety of parameters including physical assessment, history, anthropometric measurements and laboratory tests (Hasse, 2001). This method has been used in subjects who were followed for four years. During the first year, follow-up visits occurred once a month and they included evaluation of anthropometric measurements, body composition, biochemical parameters and dietary records; afterwards the body weight, the dietary habits, the physical activity level and the biochemical parameters were collected on the phone once a year for three years (Guida et al., 2009).

Various parameters are analyzed in the nutritional status assessment (Sirvent & Garrido, 2009).

2.1 Personal interview

The personal interview is essential to review and investigate certain aspects which may have direct bearing on the dietary pattern. Some key items to be considered are discussed in this paragraph.

In relation to food intake, it is necessary to find out the usual pattern (quantity, quality and distribution of food intake) in the last days, weeks or months. The assessment is directed at whether the intake meets minimum requirements of adequacy and variety. Related to food intake is the appetite, from which we can detect the presence of eating disorders and likely food intolerances, and delve into the personal history of diseases that alter appetite.

From a functional perspective it is necessary to inquire about ability to swallow and on digestive function and autonomy which enables food intake. It is also interesting to know more about chewing and swallowing patterns, and dental status. Reports on the presence of diarrhea, constipation, vomiting and intolerance in general should be included, and the degree of independence and autonomy of the person in relation to feeding should be checked.

Finally, we must-take into account all the circumstances which may influence and modify eating habits or energy expenditure, like family relationships, group memberships, special diets, type and frequency of physical activity, etc.

2.2 Physical inspection

Most important items when assessing physical condition are hydration, weight aspect, awareness and autonomy. These parameters influence the ability to feed , body temperature, colour of skin and mucous and should be considered as merely indicative. This should be complemented by biochemical data, anthropometric and dietary history of the subject.

2.3 Body composition

Provides information on the percentages of muscle, fat or bone. There are different methods: chemical techniques, electrical bioimpedance and anthropometry, among others. The anthropometric measurements and bioimpedance are widely used non invasive techniques.

2.3.1 Chemical techniques

Measurements of chemical techniques include creatinine and 3-methylhistidine. In relation to the first technique, the total plasma creatinine concentration is used for determining muscle mass, assuming that the creatinine is 98% in muscle tissue and 1 mg of creatinine equivalent to 0.88 kg of muscle. This technique only provides data on muscle mass, does not evaluate other parameters of body composition and has a number of drawbacks. The 3-methylhistidine is also used for determining muscle mass. Generally this shows the same disadvantages as the previous determination and we must add the complexity of the analysis and high cost.

2.3.2 Bioelectrical impedance analysis

Body composition can be determined by conventional bioelectrical impedance analysis (BIA). The subject should rest in the supine position and a weak current (electric current of low voltage high frequency and intensity) is passed between two electrodes placed on one hand and another on a foot. The intensity is conducted differently from fat (it acts as insulation) than fat-free mass, where water and electrolytes are good conductors. The use of this technique has several advantages, including: its relatively low price, ease of equipment transportation and its safety.

Because BIA equations must consider age, gender, race and body habitus of the patient (Dumler, 1997), accuracy of the results also depends on the equations used to determine body composition (de Fijter et al., 1997; Pichard et al., 1999).

Although BIA has become widely available, a single-frequency test may not be valid in transplant candidates due to body fluid shifts (Hasse, 2001).

2.3.3 Anthropometric method

The anthropometric method is highly recommended for several reasons: it is simple, accurate, accessible, comfortable and economical. The reliability depends on the ability of anthropometrics and rigor in making measurements. The protocol must be standardized so that results can be compared (Sirvent & Garrido, 2009).

Nutritional anthropometry is based on the study of a number of somatic measures on proportions of the human body. The data obtained from anthropometry (weight, height, perimeter, diameters, lengths and skin folds) are further processed by application of different regression equations and statistical formulas for information on body composition.

The parameters commonly used are weight, height and body mass index. The weight is an easily obtainable and reproducible indicator of body mass. Along with weight, the height provides less sensitive information on nutritional deficiencies. However, both parameters can be obtained on body mass index, also known as Quetelet index. In particular, BMI is defined by body weight in kilograms divided by the square of body height in metres.

Obesity is characterized by an excess of body fat. Several methods have been introduced to quantify obesity. The most common are measurement of body fat by the use of bioelectrical impedance techniques and measurements of body density by weighing subjects underwater and subsequent calculation of fat mass (Flier, 2001). As it is difficult to ascertain the exact amount of body fat, a number of markers have been development to quantify obesity.

BMI is the most widely used parameter for characterization of abnormalities of body weight (Kahn et al., 2006). The recommended classification for BMI adopted by the Expert Panel on the Identification, Evaluation and Treatment of Overweight and Obesity in Adults, and endorsed by the National Institute of Health and the WHO is: BMI<18.5 (underweight), 18.5 to 24.99 (normal weight), 25 to 29.99 (overweight), 30 to 34.99 (obesity class I), 35 t0 39.99 (obesity class II) and ≥ 40 (obesity class III) (National Heart, Lung and Blood Institute, 1998).

BMI at the time of transplant is an important predictor of post transplant outcomes, including survival, perioperative morbidity, post transplant cardiovascular comorbities, long-term complications of transplantation and survival on the waiting list. HT recipients across a broad range of BMI (including normal, overweight and obesity I subgroups) achieved good long-term post transplant outcomes. However, recipients at the extremes (e.g. underweight and obesity II/III) have significantly higher morbidity and mortality compared with other groups. This diminished survival in the underweight (BMI<18,5) group resulted from excess morbidity in the first year post transplantation. However, with correction of their heart failure and subsequent reversal of their cachectis state, their risk of death along with the mean BMI, normalized after the initial post transplant period. Obesity II/III (BMI>35) was also associated with diminished survival, however, this appears to result from higher morbidity and mortality over the long-term (Russo et al., 2010).

In cardiac surgery patients, a low BMI increased the relative hazard for death and low S-album increased the risk for infection. Rapp-Kesek et al. suggest that these parameters provide useful information in the preoperative evaluation (Rapp-Kesek et al., 2004).

On the other hand, skin folds and body parameters are widely used (Sirvent & Garrido, 2009).

In this sense, the most common measures used are Triceps skin fold (PT), Circular circumference of the arm (CB) and Arm muscle circumference (AMC). PT allows us to assess fat mass. It is expressed in mm, and its measurement is made with a calliper at the midpoint between the acromion and the olecranon. On the other hand, CB provides information about the total mass and is measured with a tape measure midway between the acromion and the olecranon and expressed in cm. Last, AMC is used to assess muscle mass. It is expressed in cm and is calculated: CMB (cm) = CB (cm) -0.314 x PT (mm).

2.3.4 Biochemical parameters

Biochemical parameters make possible obtaining more information on nutritional status. They are (among others):

- Albumin is one of the most used. This protein has a long half life (18-20 days), so their determination is a few sensitive markers in recent nutritional disorders. Instead it may be useful to assess long and serious situations of malnutrition. The normal concentration for adults is ≥ 3.5 g/dl. Hypoalbuminemia presents low risk values between 2.8 and 3.4 g/dl and hypoalbuminemia high-risk values are below 2.8 g/dl.
- Transferring is also widely used. It has a shorter half life between 8 and 10 days. Its main function is iron transport functions. It is more sensitive than albumin to nutritional changes and responds more quickly to changes in protein status. Normal levels are between 150 and 200 mg/dl. It considers moderate deficiency between 100 and 150 mg/dl and severe deficiency below 100 mg/dl.
- Prealbumin is a transport protein with a half life of 2 days. It decreases rapidly when calorific intake or protein is low and responds very quickly to nutritional rehabilitation. Normal values are between 10 and 40 mg/dl.
- Retinol transport protein has a very short half life of approximately 12 hours. Its values are normal at 7.6 mg/dl. Sensitivity to protein-energy deprivation is high, but lacks (as prealbumin) diagnostic specificity due to the impact of other processes on its levels.
- Fibronectin. Studies have shown low levels in situations of fasting and acute protein-energy malnutrition. Its normalization with nutritional rehabilitation is rapid. Normal values are around 169 mg/ml.
- Nitrogen balance provides information on the protein reserve. We reserve its use to situations where we want to have guidance on protein balance in a given time.
- Lymphocyte count, based on an adequate supply of energy and protein is essential for maintaining normal immune function. The drawbacks are its low specificity because it can be altered by multiple factors and the other limitation is that only the lymphocyte count is altered in situations when malnutrition is established.

Finally, we mention the existence of other parameters used in specific situations, such as vitamin A, vitamin E and so on. Measurement and interpretation of waist circumference and fasting triglycerides could be used among heart transplant patients for early identification of men characterized by the presence of elevated fasting insulin and apolipoprotein B concentration, and small LDL particles. The presence of the atherogenic metabolic triad identifies patients at high risk of coronary artery disease, even in the heart transplant population (Sénéchal et al., 2005).

3. Nutritional intervention

Nutrition is extremely important in the care of patients undergoing transplantation (Helton, 2001). Following an appropriate and strict dietary regimen after the HT reduces risk factors and should be considered seriously (Guida et al., 2009).

During the acute post transplant phase, adequate nutrition is required to help prevent infection, promote wound healing, support metabolic demands, replenish lost stores and perhaps mediate the immune response (Hasse, 2001).

The HT recipient must have two main dietary goals: a healthy and balanced diet (to provide all the necessary nutrients and avoid new heart attacks) and to maintain strict hygiene measures to reduce germs in food (Casado, 2005).

With regard to the rules of food hygiene, there are a number of recommendations among which are: do not take raw food during the first six months post transplant (considered the highest risk); casseroles prepared at home, if not eaten immediately after cooking, should be kept in the fridge covered and consumed within 24 hours; do not add anything raw to the preparation; it is preferable to keep sauces separate (Casado, 2005).

A diet of cardiovascular protection should include the following considerations about certain parameters:

3.1 Overweight

Some investigators have described excessive weight gain following cardiac transplant (Baker et al., 1992; Johnson et al., 2002; Keteyian et al., 1992; Lake et al., 1993). On average these patients gain approximately 10 kg within the first year after the procedure. This weight gain increases the risk of secondary diseases (i.e. hypertension, diabetes and dislipemias) (Williams, 2006).

Patients who were underweight or obese at one year post transplant were at greater risk of rejection over time than patients who were of normal weight or overweight. Post transplant cachexia and obesity are risk factors for poor clinical outcomes after heart transplantation. Grady et al. found that risk factors for increased body weight at one year after heart transplantation included both demographic factors (BMI at the time of transplant, younger age, black race) and clinical variables (etiology of heart disease, immunosuppression) (Grady, 2005).

After HT, regular weight-bearing and muscle-strengthening exercise should be encouraged to reduce the risk of falls and fractures, and to increase bone density. Lifestyle modifications, including weight loss, low-sodium diet and exercise are appropriate adjuncts to facilitate control of blood pressure in HT recipients (Costanzo et al., 2010). The clinicians may assist patients to make changes in their post transplant lifestyle to return to a normal body weight.

Guida et al. showed the efficacy of dietary intervention to obtain an early and late weight and metabolic control after HT. All subjects received a dietary plan that was elaborated to fit an energy intake ≥ 25 Kcal/Kg/Ideal Body Weight/day, with 55% of carbohydrates, 15% of protein and 30% of total fat (fatty acids <10% of calories and dietary cholesterol <300 mg/d according the American Heart Association step one diet guidelines) (The Expert Panel, 1988). The patients were prescribed low-salt food in order not to exceed sodium content of 1.5 g/d and they were asked to limit the amount of additional salt to 3 g/d. In this diet plan all subjects were encouraged to increase their physical activity level up to 30 min/d three times a week and they were strongly recommended to modify some of their habits (Guida et al., 2009).

To reach this goal it is indispensable to carry out an early and comprehensive programme providing a plan of nutritional interventions, education and lifestyle counselling. They demonstrated that dietary compliance is helpful to get a good early and late control in weight and metabolic parameters, both in subjects enrolled during the first year from the transplant and after the first year from the transplant, even if high doses of immunosuppressive therapy are used. The beneficial effects of this intervention are still maintained after a 48-month follow-up period (Guida et al., 2009).

Incorporation of a weight loss plan, including diet, exercise and psychologic interventions into the discharge process with subsequent outpatient follow-up is recommended. The psychological interventions are often incorporated into a comprehensive weight loss programme (Grady, 2005).

The scientific literature shows different mood disorders in both the situation prior to transplantation and thereafter; the most common that have been tested are the anxiety disorders, depression and post traumatic stress disorder (Perez San Gregorio et al., 2005; Spaderna et al., 2007) and they have been found to adversely affect the ability to accept the new organ.

This negative emotion affects different areas of the daily life of transplant patients, including nutritional status, either with a decreased or increased appetite, and consequently a loss or weight gain, which is contraindicated in patients transplanted.

Although a variety of weight loss programmes exist, it may be beneficial to consider weight loss plans that are individualized and tailored to incorporate the patient's clinical status, age, cultural background, dietary preferences, exercise history, socio-economic and behavioural factors etc. Many patients also have established patterns of cooking and eating based on cultural background (Grady, 2005).

Moreover, the goal of a dietary intervention should be to optimize the nutritional status and to preserve the long-term renal function by avoiding unnecessary protein loads (Al et al., 2005).

With respect to lipid metabolism, the increase in body weight is correlated with the increase in serum lipid level during the first year after the transplant (Grady et al., 1991; Keogh et al., 1988), whereas a decrease in body weight or energy intake is effective to reduce blood cholesterol level (Kannel et al., 1979; Nichols et al., 1976; Kromhout, 1983).

3.2 Malnutrition

Harrison et al. defined malnutrition as midarm muscle circumference and triceps skin fold measurement <25th percentile (Harrison et al., 1997). The malnutrition diagnosed by subjective and objective nutrition assessment parameters is common in solid organ transplant recipients and leads to increased morbidity and mortality (Helton, 2001).
Because malnutrition is a marker of worsening heart failure (Anker et al., 1997) and is a known risk factor for poor outcomes after surgery (Buzby et al., 1980; Rady et al., 1997) low BMI may in fact be a stronger predictor of poor outcomes than obesity. The BMI is potentially modifiable through medical management and/or lifestyle changes (Russo et al., 2010).

Patients with chronic heart failure are often malnourished as a result of maldigestion, malabsorption and poor nutrient assimilation. This is compounded by the fact that many of these patients have a prolonged catabolic state characterized by increased energy expenditure coupled with anorexia and inadequate dietary intake.

Malnourished patients undergoing transplantation have increased morbidity and mortality, and increased overall hospital charges. Patients surviving transplantation have altered lipid and fat metabolism, and problems with obesity and accelerated atherosclerosis leading to cardiovascular death (Helton, 2001).

3.3 Dyslipidemia

Dyslipidemia is common after cardiac transplantation. Multiple factors in transplant recipients promote dyslipemia: inappropriate diet in combination with reduced physical activity, immunosuppression with cyclosporine and steroids, anti-hypertensive agents and concomitant conditions, such as diabetes, obesity, age and male gender. Total and low-density lipoprotein (LDL) cholesterol are prominent risk factors for major progression of CAV disease (Pethig et al., 2000).

To accommodate the lipid profile the following is recommended: a cholesterol intake below 300 mg per day, to limit total dietary fat to less than 30% of total calories, to limit saturated fats to less than 10% of total calories, to increase mono- and polyunsaturated fat (the latter about 7% of total calories) (Casado, 2005).

In recent years the benefit of certain food components has been referenced. Phytosterol, plant stanol and sterol esters, reduce serum cholesterol by inhibition of cholesterol absorption. Substitution of part of the daily fat intake with stanol ester margarine has been shown to reduce serum cholesterol by 10.2% and LDL cholesterol by 14% after one year (Miettinen et al., 1995).

Margarine containing stanol/sterol esters is a safe, simple and efficient way to reduce total LDL cholesterol in patients after cardiac transplantation. The tolerance of the margarine containing stanol or sterol esters is good. It is possible to reduce the dose of statins while maintaining LDL cholesterol at <115 mg/dl (Vorlat et al., 2003). The concomitant use of statins and stanol esters has shown additional lipid-lowering effects (Blair et al., 2000).

Phytosterol therapy produces an average 10-11% reduction in LDL cholesterol concentration, but it is unknown whether this effect persists beyond two years. Phytosterol products are well tolerated and have few drug interactions, but their long-term safety has not been established. Current evidence is sufficient to recommend phytosterol for lowering LDL cholesterol in adults (Malinowski & Gehret, 2010).

On the other hand, ω-3 fatty acids have been studied in cardiac transplant recipients treated with cyclosporine and have been found to have beneficial effects on hypertension (Andreassen et al., 1997; Holm et al., 2001) and coronary endothelial function (Fleischhauer et al., 1993). They may also be added to statin therapy in cardiac transplant recipients with persistent hypertriglyceridemia. An ω-3 fish oil preparation consisting of 80% ω-3 polyunsaturated fatty acids (44% eicosapentaenoic acid and 36% dehydroacetic acid) when used with simvastatin has been shown to reduce triglyceride levels by an additional 20-30% (Durrington et al., 2001). When triglyceride levels are >200 mg/dl after LDL-lowering therapy, a trial of an ω-3 concentrate or fish oil (which usually contains approximately 35% ω-3 polyunsaturated fatty acids) is reasonable because of the potential benefits and favourable safety profile (Bilchick et al., 2004).

3.4 Beneficial effects of certain nutrients

There are investigations that demonstrate that single nutrients, such as arginine, ω-3 fatty acids and pyruvate, and the fasted and post absorptive state can dramatically alter the short and long-term function of transplanted organs (Helton, 2001).

Nutrition also may be used to help treat symptoms of end-stage organ failure. For example, an increased intake of calories and protein should help deter fat and muscle loss. Fluid retention can be treated with dietary sodium restriction. Branched-chain amino acid-enhanced formulas may be helpful for patients with intractable hepatic encephalopathy. Adequate intake of iron, folic acid and B vitamins can prevent or treat anaemia. Medium-chain triglyceride supplementation may be useful when steatorrhea and long-chain fat malabsorption are present (Hasse, 2001).

3.4.1 Calcium and vitamin D

Calcium and vitamin D are necessary when patients have osteoporosis or renal osteodystrophy (Hasse, 2001). Magnesium depletion (hypomagnesemia has been documented in cardiac transplant recipients) which may be the results of diuretic therapy, has been implicated as a risk factor for osteoporosis.

After transplantation, there is further acceleration in bone loss. Factors associated with congestive heart failure that may contribute to bone loss include cardiac cachexia, reduced exercise or immobilisation, smoking, alcohol abuse, low calcium intake, heparine administration and loop diuretics (Pisani & Mullen, 2002). Vitamin D deficiency is significantly more common in the patients with more severe heart failure (Rodino & Shane, 1998).

Optimal treatment of osteoporosis requires adequate calcium and vitamin D intake. The Institute of Medicine recommends calcium intakes of 1000 to 1500 mg/d (depending on age and menopausal status) for adults (NIH, 2001) and vitamin D (400-1000 IU, or as necessary to maintain serum 25-hydroxyvitamin D levels above 30 mg/ml= 75 nmol/L) (Costanzo et al., 2010). Of note, bone loss occurs despite supplementation with vitamin D and calcium

(Shane et al., 1997). The use of calcium and vitamin D supplements, although recommended, is inadequate for the prevention of bone loss and complications such as vertebral fractures (Pisani & Mullen, 2002).

3.4.2 Folic acid

The aminoacid homocysteine has recently been identified as a risk factor for native coronary artery disease (Welch et al., 1997) and even mild to moderate hyperhomocysteinemia is associated with premature vascular disease (Kark et al., 1999). Growing evidence suggests that elevated total plasma homocysteine levels (tHCY) are associated with CAV following heart transplantation (Kutschka et al., 2001).

The homeostasis of homocysteine is altered in solid organ transplant recipients and may be partially caused by cyclosporine. The cyclosporine may be associated with secondary hyperhomocysteinemia by inducing renal insufficiency.

Homocysteine is formed by the transmethylation of methionine. Its catabolim is either through a folate-cobalamin dependent remethylation pathway catalyzed by methionine synthase, or by transsulfuration by cystationine-synthasa, a vitamin B6-dependent enzyme (Chan, 2001).

Beside parameters like age (Kark et al., 1999), sex (Selhub et al., 1999), genetic determination (Deloughery et al., 1996) and renal function (Moustapha et al., 1998) are influenced by dietary intake of vitamins B6, B12 and folic acid (Selhub et al., 1999; Verhoef et al., 1996). Hyperhomocysteinemia as well as deficiencies in folate and vitamin B6 are common in HT recipients, especially in older individuals and patients with renal insufficiency (Kutschka et al., 2001).

Folic acid supplementation (5 mg per day) provides a simple and effective measure to lower elevated tHCY concentrations without side effects (Kutschka et al., 2001, Chan, 2001).

3.4.3 L-Arginine

Endothelial dysfunction is associated with the decreased exercise capacity observed in HT recipients. L-Arginine supplementation (LAS) increases nitric oxide (NO) and decreases endothelin-1 plasma concentrations, thereby improving endothelial function and exercise capacity in heart failure or HT patients (Doutreleau et al., 2004; Rector et al., 1996).

The NO/endothelin ratio significantly increases after chronic LAS, suggesting that the beneficial effects of L-Arginine (amino acid precursor of NO production) on the exercise capacity of patients after an HT might, at least partly, be related to an improvement in skeletal muscle vasodilatation and oxygen delivery, and extraction during exercise as suggested by the significant increase in the oxygen pulse after LAS. This pilot study provides support that oral LAS may be a useful adjuvant therapy to improve the quality of life and exercise tolerance in HT recipients (Doutreleau et al., 2010). The L-Arginine-NO pathway has been recognized to play critical roles during infection, inflammation, organ injury and transplant rejection (Helton, 2001).

These dietary interventions, when used in combination with other therapies, may improve the quality of life of patients (Hasse, 2001).

3.5 Side effects of cyclosporine

Cyclosporine has significant effects on the metabolism and disposition of several biomolecules. Hyperglycemia, hypercholesterolemia and electrolyte disturbances are a few of its common side effects. Hyperkalemia (cyclosporine has a direct effect on the renin-angiotensin-aldosterone system which further worsens potassium homeostasis [Bantle et al., 1985]) and hypomagnesemia are the two most frequently observed electrolyte disorders caused by this calcineurin inhibitor.

Patients taking cyclosporine should be educated on their dietary potassium intake (the hypertension is another common side effect of cyclosporine). Most patients will subsequently require oral supplementation of magnesium to maintain a normo-magnesic state and the chronic hypomagnesemia may affect parathyroid function and rennin activity (Ichihara et al., 1993; Mori et al., 1992; Navarro et al., 1999). The altered parathyroid hormone activity can have a secondary effect on calcium and vitamin D disposition, and may indirectly contribute to post transplant osteoporosis (Grenet et al., 2000; Thiébaud et al., 1996).

3.6 Mediterranean diet

It has been suggested that the healthy effects of the Mediterranean diet observed in epidemiologic studies are exerted partly through plausible mechanisms: improved lipid profiles (Bemelmans et al., 2002; Zambón et al., 2000) and reductions in blood pressure (Perona et al., 2004) , insulin resistance and systemic markers of inflammation (Chrysohoou et al., 2004; Esposito et al., 2004). These beneficial effects on surrogate markers of cardiovascular risk add biological plausibility to the epidemiologic evidence that supports the suggested protective effects of the Mediterranean diet (Estruch et al., 2006). Moreover, the Mediterranean diet could protect against the development of coronary heart disease, not only because of its beneficial role regarding cardiovascular risk factors, but also due to a possible effect on body weight and obesity (Kastorini et al., 2010).

4. Drug-nutrient interaction

HT recipients are polymedicated patients; they use multiple medications to manage graft rejection, opportunistic infections and other associated complications. This patient population has a very high risk of drug-nutrient interactions (Chan, 2006). In some cases, the interactions are not identified until serious adverse events have occurred.

The consequences of unrecognized and unmanaged drug-nutrient interactions in the transplant recipient can be very serious and these adverse outcomes represent important contributing factors to post transplant morbidity and mortality (Chan, 2001).

Drug-nutrient interactions can significantly affect the availability and potency of immunosuppressive therapy. Alterations in food intake, inadequate digestion and these interactions can lead to changes in the pharmacokinetics of immunosuppressive drugs leading to either toxicity or organ rejection as a result of inadequate blood drug levels (Helton, 2001).

Drugs have the potential to interact with nutrients, which could lead to the reduced therapeutic efficacy of the drug, nutritional risk or increased adverse effects of the drug.

Food-drug interactions are defined as alterations of pharmacokinetics or pharmacodynamics of a drug or nutritional element, or a compromise in nutritional status as a result of the addition of a drug. Nutrient-drug interactions can result in two clinical effects: either a decreased bioavailability of a drug, which predisposes to treatment failure, or an increased bioavailability, which increases the risk of adverse events and may even precipitate toxicities (Genser, 2008).

On the other hand, medications can lead to altered food choices. Many drugs are reported to directly affect the sense of taste and smell, and some drugs themselves have an unpleasant taste that might interfere with food intake (Brownie, 2006).

The evidence that water-soluble vitamin E interacts with orally administered cyclosporine is quite convincing. This interaction has only been observed with water-soluble formulation of vitamin E. Further investigations using different dosage forms of vitamin E are necessary. Grapefruit juice-drug interactions represent some of the most significant examples of drug-nutrient interactions. When a single dose of cyclosporine was taken with 200 mL of grapefruit juice, its absorption was increased. The reported increase in bioavailability of cyclosporine ranged from 17% to 63% (Chan, 2001).

Other drugs with increased absorption when taken with grapefruit juice are atorvastatin and sertralin (Chan, 2006).

5. Conclusion

It is necessary to make more efforts in studying the metabolic syndrome in transplant patients and how this syndrome can affect the transplanted graft.

There are still many doubts about the interactions between different drugs used, nutrients and other substances in the diet. Moreover, further studies are needed to provide information on the potential benefit that some types of diet (such as the Mediterranean), antioxidants or other molecules present in the diet can contribute to the benefit of patients. Moreover, not only is it important to know that various substances can be beneficial, it is also important to know the amount we can use.

6. References

Al, Z.; Abbas, S.; Moore, E.; Diallo, O.; Hauptman, PJ. & Bastani B. (2005). The natural history of renal function following orthotopic heart transplant. *Clin Transplant*. Vol. 19, No. 5, (Oct 2005), pp. 683-689.

Almenar, ML.; Cardo, L.; Martínez-Dolz, C.; García-Palomar, J.; Rueda, E.; Zorio, MA.; et al. (2005). Risk factors affecting survival in heart transplant patients. *Transplantation Proceedings*, Vol. 37, (2005), pp. 4011-4013.

Andreassen, AK.; Hartmann, A.; Offstad, J.; Geiran, O.; Kvernebo, K. & Simonsen S. (1997). Hypertension prophylaxis with omega-3 fatty acids in heart transplant recipients. *J Am Coll Cardiol*. Vol. 29, No. 6, (May 1997), pp. 1324-1331.

Anker, SD.; Chua, TP.; Ponikowski, P.; Harrington, D.; Swan, JW.; Kox, WJ.; et al. (1997). Hormonal changes and catabolic/anabolic imbalance in chronic failure and their importance for cardiac cachexia. *Circulation*, Vol. 96, No. 2, (July 1997), pp. 526–534.

Anker, SD.; Ponikowski, P.; Varney, S.; Chua, TP.; Clark, AL.; Webb-Peploe, KM.; et al. (1997). Wasting as independent risk factor for mortality in chronic heart failure. *Lancet*. Vol. 349, No. 9058, (Apr 1997), pp. 1050-1053.

Baker, AM.; Levine, TB.; Goldberg, AD. & Levine AB. Natural history and predictors of obesity after orthotopic heart transplantation. *J Heart Lung Transplant*. Vol. 11, No. 6, (Nov-Dec 1992), pp. 1156-1159.

Bantle, JP.; Nath, KA.; Sutherland, DE.; Najarian, JS. & Ferris TF. (1985). Effects of cyclosporine on the renin-angiotensin-aldosterone system and potassium excretion in renal transplant recipients. *Arch Intern Med*. Vol. 145, No. 3, (Mar 1985), pp. 505-508.

Bemelmans, WJ.; Broer, J.; Feskens, EJ.; Smit, AJ.; Muskiet, FA.; Lefrandt, JD.; et al. (2002). Effect of an increased intake of alpha-linolenic acid and group nutritional education on cardiovascular risk factors: the Mediterranean Alpha-linolenic Enriched Groningen Dietary Intervention (MARGARIN) study. *Am J Clin Nutr*. Vol. 75, No. 2, (Feb 2002), pp. 221-227.

Bilchick, K.; Henrikson, C.; Skojec, D.; Kasper, E. & Blumenthal, R. (2004). Treatment of hyperlipidemia in cardiac transplant recipients. *American Heart Journal*, Vol. 148, No. 2, (August 2004), pp. 200-210.

Blair, SN.; Capuzzi, DM.; Gottlieb, SO.; Nguyen, T.; Morgan, JM. & Cater NB. (2000). Incremental reduction of serum total cholesterol and low-density lipoprotein cholesterol with the addition of plant stanol ester-containing spread to statin therapy. *Am J Cardiol*. Vol. 86, No. 1, (Jul 2000), pp. 46-52.

Brownie, S. (2006). Why are elderly individuals at risk of nutritional deficiency? *Int J Nurs Pract*. Vol. 12, No. 2, (Apr 2006), pp.110-8.

Buzby, GP.; Mullen, JL.; Matthews, DC.; Hobbs, CL. & Rosato, EF. (1980). Prognostic nutritional index in gastrointestinal surgery. *Am J Surg*. Vol. 139, No. 1, (Jan 1980), pp. 160-167.

Casado, M.J. (2005). Recomendaciones nutricionales para el paciente transplantado de corazón. *Enfermería en Cardiología*, No.34, (2005), pp. 22-24.

Costanzo, MR.; Dipchand, A.; Starling, R.; Taylor, D.; Meiser, B.; Webber, S.; et al. (2010). The International Society of Heart and Lung Transplantation Guidelines for the care of heart transplant recipients. *The Journal of Heart and Lung Transplantation*, Vol. 29, No. 8, (August 2010), pp. 914-956.

Chan, LN. (2001). Drug-nutrient interactions in transplant recipients. *J Parenter Enteral Nutr*. Vol. 25, No. 3, (May-Jun 2001), pp. 132-141.

Chan, LN. (2006). Drug-Nutrient Interactions. In: Shils, ME.; Shike, M.; Ross, AC.; Caballero, B.; Cousins, RJ. (eds): *Modern Nutrition in Health and Disease.* Baltimore, Lippincott Williams & Wilkins, 2006, pp. 1540–1553.

Chrysohoou, C.; Panagiotakos, DB.; Pitsavos, C.; Das, UN. & Stefanadis, C. (2004). Adherence to the Mediterranean diet attenuates inflammation and coagulation process in healthy adults: The ATTICA Study. *J Am Coll Cardiol*. Vol. 44, No. 1, (Jul 2004), pp. 152-158.

de Fijter, WM.; de Fijter, CW.; Oe, PL.; ter Wee, PM. & Donker, AJ. (1997). Assessment of total body water and lean body mass from anthropometry, Watson formula, creatinine kinetics and body electrical impedance compared with antipyrine kinetics in peritoneal dialysis patients. *Nephrol Dial Transplant*. Vol. 12, No. 1, (Jan 1997), pp. 151-156.

Deloughery, TG.; Evans, A.; Sadeghi, A.; McWilliams, J.; Henner, WD.; Taylor, LM.; et al. (1996). Common mutation in methylenetetrahydrofolate reductase. Correlation with homocysteine metabolism and late-onset vascular disease. *Circulation*. Vol. 94, No. 12, (Dec 1996), pp. 3074-3078.

Doutreleau, S.; Rouyer, O.; Di Marco, P.; Lonsdorfer, E.; Richard, R.; Piquard, F.; et al. (2010). L-arginine supplementation improves exercise capacity after a heart transplant. *Am J Clin Nutr*. Vol. 91, No. 5, (May 2010), pp. 1261-1267.

Doutreleau, S.; Piquard, F. ; Lonsdorfer, E. ; Rouyer, O. ; Lampert, E. ; Mettauer, B. ; et al. (2004). Improving exercise capacity, 6 wk training tends to reduce circulating endothelin after heart transplantation. *Clin Transplant*. Vol. 18, No. 6, (Dec 2004), pp. 672-675.

Dumler, F. (1997). Use of bioelectric impedance analysis and dual-energy X-ray absorptiometry for monitoring the nutritional status of dialysis patients. *ASAIO J*. Vol. 43, No. 3, (May-Jun 1997), pp. 256-260.

Durrington, PN.; Bhatnagar, D.; Mackness, MI.; Morgan, J.; Julier, K.; Khan, MA.; et al. (2001). An omega-3 polyunsaturated fatty acid concentrate administered for one year decreased triglycerides in simvastatin treated patients with coronary heart disease and persisting hypertriglyceridaemia. *Heart*. Vol. 85, No. 5, (May 2001), pp. 544-548.

Epstein, S.; Shane, E. & Bilezikian J. Organ transplantation and osteoporosis. (1995). *Curr Opin Rheumatol*, Vol. 7, No. 3, (May 1995), pp. 255–261.

Epstein, S. & Shane, E. (1996). Post transplant bone disease: the role of immunosuppressive agents on the skeleton. *J Bone Miner Res*. Vol. 11. (1996), pp. 1-7.

Esposito, K.; Marfella, R.; Ciotola, M.; Di Palo, C.; Giugliano, F.; Giugliano, G.; et al. (2004). Effect of a Mediterranean-style diet on endothelial dysfunction and markers of vascular inflammation in the metabolic syndrome: a randomized trial. *JAMA*. Vol. 292, No. 12, (Sep 2004), pp. 1440-1446.

Estruch, R.; Martínez-González, MA.; Corella, D.; Salas-Salvadó, J.; Ruiz-Gutiérrez, V.; Covas, MI.; et al. (2006). Effects of a Mediterranean-style diet on cardiovascular risk factors: a randomized trial. *Ann Intern Med*. Vol. 145, No. 1, (Jul 2006), pp. 1-11.

Evangelista, LS.; Dracup, K.; Doering, L.; Moser, DK. & Kobashigawa, J. (2005). Physical activity patterns in heart transplant women. *J Cardiovasc Nurs*, Vol. 20, No. 5, (Sept-Oct 2005), pp. 334-339.

Flattery, MP.; Salyer, J.; Maltby, MC.; Joyner, PL. & Elswick, RK. (2006). Lifestyle and health status differ over time in long-term heart transplant recipients. *Prog Transplant*, Vol. 16, No. 3, (September 2006), pp. 232-238.

Fleischhauer, FJ.; Yan, WD. & Fischell TA. (1993). Fish oil improves endothelium-dependent coronary vasodilation in heart transplant recipients. *J Am Coll Cardiol*. Vol. 21, No. 4, (Mar 1993), pp. 982-989.

Flier, JS. (2001). Obesity - definition and measurement. In: Braunwald, E.; Fauci, AS.; Kasper, D.; Hauser, S.; Jameson, J. & Stone, R. eds. *Harrison's Principles of Internal Medicine*, 15th edn. New York; St Louis, MO: McGraw-Hill Book Company, 2001.

Genser, D. (2008). Food and drug interaction: consequences for the nutrition/health status. *Ann Nutr Metab*. Vol. 52, Suppl 1, (2008), pp. 29-32.

Glendenning, P.; Kent, GN.; Adler, BD.; Matz, L.; Watson, I.; O'Driscoll, GJ.; et al. (1999). High prevalence of osteoporosis in cardiac transplant recipients and discordance between biochemical turnover markers and bone histomorphometry. *Clin Endocrinol*. Vol. 50, No.3, (Mar 1999), pp.347–355.

Grady, KL.; Naftel, D.; Pamboukian, SV.; Frazier, OH.; Hauptman, P.; Herre, J.; et al. (2005). Post-operative obesity and cachexia are risk factors for morbidity and mortality after heart transplant: multi-institutional study of post-operative weight change. *J Heart Lung Transplant.* Vol. 24, No. 9, (Sep 2005), pp. 1424-1430.

Grady, KL.; Costanzo-Nordin, MR.; Herold, LS.; Sriniavasan, S. & Pifarre, R. (1991). Obesity and hyperlipidemia after heart transplantation. *J Heart Lung Transplant.* Vol. 10, No.3, (May-Jun 1991), pp. 449-454.

Grenet, O.; Bobadilla, M.; Chibout, SD. & Steiner S. Evidence for the impairment of the vitamin D activation pathway by cyclosporine A. *Biochem Pharmacol.* Vol. 59, No. 3, (Feb 2000), pp. 267-272.

Guida, B.; Perrino, NR.; Laccetti, R.; Trio, R.; Nastasi, A.; Pesola, D.; et al. (2009). Role of dietary intervention and nutritional follow-up in heart transplant recipients. *Clin Transplant.* Vol. 23. No. 1, (Jan-Feb 2009), pp. 101-107.

Harrison, J.; McKiernan, J. & Neuberger JM. (1997). A prospective study on the effect of recipient nutritional status on outcome in liver transplantation. *Transpl Int.* Vol. 10, No. 5, (1997), pp. 369-374.

Hasse, J. (2001). Nutrition assessment and support of organ transplants recipients. *Journal of Parenteral and Enteral Nutrition,* Vol. 25, No. 3, (May/Jun 2001), pp. 120-131.

Helton, W. (2001). The A.S.P.E.N. Research Workshop Nutrition Support in Transplantation *Journal of Parenteral and Enteral Nutrition,* Vol. 25, No. 3, (May/Jun 2001), pp. 111-113.

Henderson, NK.; Sambrook, PN.; Kelly, PJ.; Macdonald, P.; Keogh, AM.; Spratt, P.; et al. (1995). Bone mineral loss and recovery after cardiac transplantation. *Lancet.* Vol. 346, No. 8979, (Sep 1995), pp. 905.

Holm, T.; Andreassen, AK.; Aukrust, P.; Andersen, K.; Geiran, OR.; Kjekshus, J.; et al. (2001). Omega-3 fatty acids improve blood pressure control and preserve renal function in hypertensive heart transplant recipients. *Eur Heart J.* Vol. 22, No. 5, (Mar 2001), pp. 428-436.

Hosenpud, J.; Bennett, L.; , Keck, B.; Fiol, B.; Boucek, M. & Novick R. (1998). The Registry of the International Society for Heart and Lung Transplantation: fifteenth official report 1998. *J Heart Lung Transplant,* Vol. 17, (1998), pp. 656–668.

Ichihara, A.; Suzuki, H. & Saruta, T. (1993). Effects of magnesium on the renin-angiotensin-aldosterone system in human subjects. *J Lab Clin Med.* Vol. 122, No. 4, (Oct 1993), pp. 432-440.

Johnson, DW.; Isbel, NM.; Brown, AM.; Kay, TD.; Franzen, K.; Hawley, CM.; et al. (2002). The effect of obesity on renal transplant outcomes. *Transplantation.* Vol. 74, No. 5, (Sep 2002), pp. 675-681.

Kahn, BB. & Flier, JS. (2000). Obesity and insulin resistance. *J Clin Invest.* Vol. 106, No. 4, (Aug 2000), pp. 473-481.

Kahn, J.; Rehak, P.; Schweiger, M.; Wasler, A.; Wascher, T.; Tscheliessnigg, KH.; et al. (2006). The impact of overweight on the development of diabetes after heart transplantation. *Clin Transplant.* Vol. 20, No. 1, (Jan-Feb 2006), pp. 62-66.

Kannel, WB.; Gordon, T. & Castelli, WP. (1979). Obesity, lipids and glucose intolerance. The Framingham Study. *Am J Clin Nutr.* Vol. 32, No. 6, (Jun 1979), pp. 1238-1245.

Kark, JD.; Selhub, J.; Adler, B.; Gofin, J.; Abramson, JH.; Friedman, G.; et al. (1999). Nonfasting plasma total homocysteine level and mortality in middle-aged and elderly men and women in Jerusalem. *Ann Intern Med.* Vol. 131, No. 5, (Sep 1999), pp. 321-330.

Kastorini, CM.; Milionis, HJ.; Goudevenos, JA. & Panagiotakos, DB. (2010). Mediterranean diet and coronary heart disease: is obesity a link? - A systematic review. *Nutr Metab Cardiovasc Dis*. Vol. 20, No. 7, (Sep 2010), pp. 536-551.

Kemna, MS.; Valentine, HA.; Hunt, SA.; Schoeder, JS.; Chen, YDI. & Reaven GR. (1994). Metabolic risk factors for atherosclerosis in heart transplant recipients. *Am Heart J*, Vol. 128, No. 1, (Jul 1994), pp. 68–72.

Keogh, A.; Simons, L.; Spratt, P.; Esmore, D.; Chang, V.; Hickie, J.; et al. (1988). Hyperlipidemia after heart transplantation. *J Heart Transplant*. Vol. 7, No. 3, (May-Jun 1988), pp. 171-175.

Keteyian, SJ.; Marks, CR.; Fedel, FJ.; Ehrman, JK.; Goslin, BR.; Connolly, AM.; et al. (1992). Assessment of body composition in heart transplant patients *Med Sci Sports Exerc*. Vol. 24, No. 2, (Feb 1992), pp. 247-252.

Kromhout, D. (1983). Body weight, diet and serum cholesterol in 871 middle-aged men during 10 years of follow-up (the Zutphen Study). *Am J Clin Nutr*. Vol. 38, No. 4, (Oct 1983), pp. 591-598.

Kutschka, I.; Pethig, K.; Strüber, M.; Dieterich, C.; Harringer, W. & Haverich, A. (2001). Homocysteine - a treatable risk factor for allograft vascular disease after heart transplantation? *J Heart Lung Transplant*. Vol. 20, No. 7, (Jul 2001), pp. 743-746.

Lake, KD.; Reutzel, TJ.; Pritzker, MR.; Jorgensen, CR. & Emery RW. (1993). The impact of steroid withdrawal on the development of lipid abnormalities and obesity in heart transplant recipients. *J Heart Lung Transplant*. Vol. 12, No. 4, (Jul-Aug 1993), pp. 580-590.

Malinowski, JM. & Gehret, MM. (2010). Phytosterols for dyslipidemia. *Am J Health Syst Pharm*. Vol. 67, No. 14, (Jul 2010), pp. 1165-1173.

Miettinen, TA.; Puska, P.; Gylling, H.; Vanhanen, H. & Vartiainen, E. (1995). Reduction of serum cholesterol with sitostanol-ester margarine in a mildly hypercholesterolemic population. *N Engl J Med*. Vol. 333, No. 20, (Nov 1995), pp. 1308-1312.

Mori, S.; Harada, S.; Okazaki, R.; Inoue, D.; Matsumoto, T. & Ogata, E. (1992). Hypomagnesemia with increased metabolism of parathyroid hormone and reduced responsiveness to calcitropic hormones. *Intern Med*. Vol. 31, No. 6, (Jun 1992), pp. 820-824.

Moustapha, A.; Naso, A.; Nahlawi, M.; Gupta, A.; Arheart, KL.; Jacobsen, DW.; et al. (1998). Prospective study of hyperhomocysteinemia as an adverse cardiovascular risk factor in end-stage renal disease. *Circulation*. Vol. 97, No. 2, (Jan 1998), pp. 138-141.

National Heart, Lung and Blood Institute. (1998). Clinical Guidelines on the Identification, Evaluation and Treatment of Overweight and Obesity in Adults. Bethesda, MD: National Heart, Lung, and Blood Institute; 1998.

Navarro, JF.; Mora, C.; Jiménez, A.; Torres, A.; Macía, M. & García, J. (1999). Relationship between serum magnesium and parathyroid hormone levels in hemodialysis patients. *Am J Kidney Dis*. Vol. 34, No. 1, (Jul 1999), pp. 43-48.

Nichols, AB. ; Ravenscroft, C.; Lamphiear, DE. & Ostrander, LD. (1976). Independence of serum lipid levels and dietary habits. The Tecumseh study. *JAMA*. Vol. 236, No. 17, (Oct 1976), pp. 1948-1953.

NIH Consensus Development Panel on Osteoporosis Prevention, Diagnosis and Therapy. (2001). Osteoporosis prevention, diagnosis and therapy. *JAMA*. Vol. 285, No. 6, (Feb 2001), pp. 785-795.

Pérez-San Gregorio, M.A.; Martín-Rodriguez, A. & Galán- Rodríguez, A. (2005). Problemas psicológicos asociados al transplante de órganos. *Int J Clin Health Psychol*, No. 5, (2005), pp.99-114.

Perona, JS.; Cañizares, J.; Montero, E.; Sánchez-Domínguez, JM.; Catalá, A. & Ruiz-Gutiérrez, V. (2004). Virgin olive oil reduces blood pressure in hypertensive elderly subjects. *Clin Nutr*. Vol. 23, No. 5, (Oct 2004), pp. 1113-1121.

Pethig, K.; Fischer, H.; Wahlers, T.; Harringer, W.; Oppelt, P. & Haverich A. (1997). odesursachen nach Herz-transplantation: Einfluß auf die klinische Langzeitbetreuung. *Z Kardiol*, Vol. 86, S3, (1997), pp. 98.

Pethig, K.; Klauss, V.; Heublein, B.; Mudra, H.; Westphal, A.; Weber, C.; et al. (2000). Progression of cardiac allograft vascular disease as assessed by serial intravascular ultrasound: correlation to immunological and non-immunological risk factors. *Heart*. Vol. 84, No. 5, (Nov 2000), pp. 494-498.

Pichard, C.; Kyle, UG. & Slosman, DO. (1999). Fat-free mass in chronic illness: comparison of bioelectrical impedance and dual-energy x-ray absorptiometry in 480 chronically ill and healthy subjects. *Nutrition*. Vol. 15, No. 9, (Sep 1999), pp. 668-676.

Pisani, B. & Mullen, GM. (2002). Prevention of osteoporosis in cardiac transplant recipients. *Curr Opin Cardiol*. Vol. 17, No. 2, (Mar 2002), pp. 160-164., pp. 473-481.

Rady, MY.; Ryan, T. & Starr, NJ. (1997). Clinical characteristics of preoperative hypoalbuminemia predict outcome of cardiovascular surgery. *J Parenter Enteral Nutr*. Vol. 21, No. 2, (Mar-Apr 1997), pp. 81-90.

Rapp-Kesek, D.; Stahle, E. & Karlsson, T. (2004). Body mass index and albumin in the preoperative evaluation of cardiac surgery patients. *Clinical Nutrition*, Vol. 23, No. 6, (Dec 2004) pp. 1398-1404.

Rector, TS.; Bank, AJ.; Mullen, KA.; Tschumperlin, LK.; Sih, R.; Pillai, K.; et al. (1996). Randomized, double-blind, placebo-controlled study of supplemental oral L-arginine in patients with heart failure. *Circulation*. Vol. 93, No. 12, (Jun 1996), pp. 2135-2141.

Reid, IR.; King, AR.; Alexander, CJ. & Ibbertson HK. (1988). Prevention of steroid-induced osteoporosis with (3-amino-1-hydroxypropylidene)-1,1-bisphosphonate (APD). *Lancet*, Vol. 331, No. 8578, (January 1988), pp. 143–146.

Rodino, M. & Shane, E. (1998). Osteoporosis after organ transplantation. *Am J Med*, Vol. 104, No. 5, (May 1998), pp. 459–469.

Russo, M.; Hong, K.; Davies, R.; Chen, J.; Mancini, D.; Oz, M.; et al. (2010). The effect of body mass index on survival following heart transplantation. Do outcomes support consensus guidelines? *Annals of Surgery*, Vol. 251, No.1, (January 2010), pp. 144-152.

Selhub, J.; Jacques, PF.; Rosenberg, IH.; Rogers, G.; Bowman, BA.; Gunter, EW.; et al. (1999). Serum total homocysteine concentrations in the third National Health and Nutrition Examination Survey (1991-1994): population reference ranges and contribution of vitamin status to high serum concentrations. *Ann Intern Med*. Vol. 131, No. 5, (Sep 1999), pp. 331-339.

Sénéchal, M.; Lemieux, I.; Beucler, I. ; Drobinski, G. ; Cormont, S. ; Dubois, M., et al. (2005). Features of the metabolic syndrome of "hypertriglyceridemic waist" and transplant coronary artery disease. *The Journal of Heart and Lung Transplantation*, Vol. 24, No. 7, (July 2005), pp. 819-826.

Shane, E. Pathogenesis and management of transplantation osteoporosis. (2000). In *Harrison's Online*, edn 15, Chap 342. Edited by Braunwald E, Fauci AS, Isselbacher, KJ, et al. New York: McGraw-Hill; 2000.

Shane, E.; Rivas, M.; McMahon, DJ.; Staron, RB.; Silverberg, SJ.; Seibel, MJ.; et al. (1997). Bone loss and turnover after cardiac transplantation. *J Clin Endocrinol Metab*. Vol. 82, No. 5, (May 1997), pp. 1497-1506.

Sirvent, J.E. & Garrido, R.P. (2009). Valoración antropomética de la composición corporal. Cineantropometria. In: Publicaciones Universidad de Alicante. Alicante, España, 2009. ISBN 978-84-9717-052-9.

Spaderna, H.; Smits, JM.; Rahmel, AO. & Weidner G. Psychosocial and behavioural factors in heart transplant candidates - an overview. *Transpl Int*. Vol. 20, No. 11, (Nov 2007), pp. 909-920.

Stempfle, HU.; Werner, C.; Echtler, S.; Wehr, U.; Rambeck, WA.; Siebert, U.; et al. (1999). Prevention of osteoporosis after cardiac transplantation: a prospective, longitudinal, randomized, double-blind trial with calcitriol. *Transplantation*, Vol. 68, No. 4, (August 1999), pp. 523-530.

The Expert Panel. (1988). National Cholesterol Education Program: report of the expert panel on the detection, evaluation and treatment of high blood cholesterol in adults. *Arch Int Med*. Vol. 148, pp. 36-69.

Thiébaud, D.; Krieg, MA.; Gillard-Berguer, D.; Jacquet, AF.; Goy, JJ. & Burckhardt P. (1996). Cyclosporine induces high bone turnover and may contribute to bone loss after heart transplantation. *Eur J Clin Invest*. Vol. 26, No. 7, (Jul 1996), pp. 549-555.

Uddén, J.; Bjo¨rntorp, P.; Arner, P.; Barkeling, B.; Meurling, L. & Ro¨ssner, S. (2003). Effects of glucocorticoids onleptin levels and eating behaviour in women. *J Intern Med*, Vol. 253, No.2, (2003), pp. 225-231.

Verhoef, P.; Stampfer, MJ.; Buring, JE.; Gaziano, JM.; Allen, RH.; Stabler, SP.; et al. (1996). Homocysteine metabolism and risk of myocardial infarction: relation with vitamins B6, B12 and folate. *Am J Epidemiol*. Vol. 143, No. 9, (May 1996), pp. 845-859.

Vorlat, A.; Conraads, VM. & Vrints, CJ. (2003). Regular use of margarine-containing stanol/sterol esters reduces total and low-density lipoprotein (LDL) cholesterol and allows reduction of statin therapy after cardiac transplantation: preliminary observations. *J Heart Lung Transplant*. Vol. 22, No. 9, (Sep 2003), pp. 1059-62.

Welch, GN.; Upchurch, G. & Loscalzo, J. (1997). Hyperhomocyst(e)inemia and atherothrombosis. *Ann N Y Acad Sci*. Vol. 811, (Apr 1997), pp. 48-58.

Williams, JJ.; Lund, LH.; LaManca, J.; Kunavarapu, C.; Cohen, DJ.; Heshka, S.; et al. (2006). Excessive weight gain in cardiac transplant recipients. *J Heart Lung Transplant*. Vol. 25, No. 1, (Jan 2006), pp. 36-41.

Zambón, D.; Sabaté, J.; Muñoz, S.; Campero, B.; Casals, E.; Merlos, M.; et al. (2000). Substituting walnuts for monounsaturated fat improves the serum lipid profile of hypercholesterolemic men and women. A randomized crossover trial. *Ann Intern Med*. Vol. 132, No. 7, (Apr 2000), pp. 538-546.

4

Physical Rehabilitation

Guilherme Veiga Guimarães, Lucas Nóbilo Pascoalino, Vitor de Oliveira Carvalho, Aline Cristina Tavares and Edimar Alcides Bocchi
Heart Failure Clinics of Heart Institute of the São Paulo University Medical School, Brazil

1. Introduction

Heart transplantation is the ultimate therapy for patients in the end stage of heart failure in order to either restore or promote patients a better functional performance (Bocchi, 2001; Guimarães, 1999).

The first heart transplant in the world was performed in 1967 and the procedure has been even more present in this area since then (Kaye, 1993). Several clinical efforts and advances were seen in the last decade in this field, with the incorporation of new surgical techniques, new immunosuppressive drugs, new diagnostic methods and approaches in the early and late postoperative. All advances were able to contribute to greater functional status and less impairment or co-morbidities.

Many different centers around in the world perform heart transplantation and, thus, are able to contribute to favorable results in terms of survival and quality of life on heart transplant recipients (Bocchi, 1999).

The practice of regular physical activity has been recommended for rehabilitation after cardiac transplantation in order to reduce and control co-morbidities (such as hypertension, diabetes, vascular disorders, mainly developed due to continuous use of immunosuppressive drugs), as well as to restore physical capacity and daily activities (Guimarães, 1999).

Nevertheless, crucial attention is needed when prescribing a physical activity program heading for heart transplant recipients, because they remain with some impairment previously to the surgery, and gain some other disabilities due to the transplantation procedure itself and due to the use of required drugs to control organ rejection.

2. Prevalence

Heart failure (HF) is the final common pathway of most diseases which affect the heart, and it is performed in these patients because of the severity and urgency of their disease (Reemtsma, 1985). Thus, **heart transplant**, or a **cardiac transplantation**, is a surgical transplant procedure performed on these patients and it is recognized as the gold standard therapy for patients facing the end stage of heart failure because there is an increased worsening imbalance between the demand for transplants and the supply of the organs in HF (Haywood, 1996).

The surgical procedure takes a working heart from a recently deceased organ donor (an allograft) and implants it into the patient (called recipient). The patient's own heart may either be removed (orthotopic transplant) or, less commonly, left in to support the donor heart (heterotopic transplant);

The cardiac transplantation contributes to a low operative mortality but an undesirable high postoperative mortality. This elucidates the fact that heart failure and the surgery represent some important current clinical challenges in healthcare and an epidemic in progress (Guimarães, 2004).

Whenever there is a careful selection for choosing the donor and recipient, there is also a significant increase in survival, exercise capacity, on return to work and quality of life of this group of patients (Banner, 1989).

From the early 80's, almost 10% of people died on the waiting list for cardiac transplantation, mostly due to sudden cardiac deaths, and the average length of time patients wait before undergoing transplantation is increasing each decade (Haywood, 1996) maybe because of the increase number of patients suffering from HF and the improvement of its palliative treatment (Guimarães, 2004).

Heart transplantation has evolved and long term survival is expected for most heart transplant recipient because of the improvements in organ preservation, surgery and immunosuppressive drug management, and physical rehabilitation.

3. Pathophysiology

In general, heart transplant surgery has become an effective therapeutic option in the management of end stage heart disease because it is able to restore physical function because the new heart doesn't have the limitations the old heart had.

There is an association of better left ventricular function one year after cardiac transplant operation with donor-related factors (donor age and sex, ischemia time), and with recipient-related factors (recipient age and sex, frequency of acute rejection), type of immunosuppressant drug, and frequency of hypertension (Reid, 1988).

However, the procedure itself promotes complete organ denervation by the postganglionic neural axons section. During heart transplant surgery, the atria of both, the giver and the receiver are sutured together (el-Gamel, 1998). The original sinoatrial node remains innervated, the vagus nerve is severed during the operation, but the electrical impulses generated by it cannot cross over the suture line.

Because the sinoatrial node of the transplanted heart, which determines heart rate (HR) is totally denervated, this neural section may be responsible for either a delay or an unsatisfactory autonomic response (Guimarães, 1999), which will depend mostly on circulating catecholamines to stimulate the heart (Kaye, 1977) unless nerve regrowth occurs.

Therefore, the absence of afferent neural control of heart rate leaves the heart under the influence of hormones in addition to internal control. The lack of neural signals to the sinoatrial node is indicated by the reduced maximal HR, heart rate variability, as well as changes in the HR response during exercise (Di Rienzo, 2001) and during change of posture (Doering, 1996).

The surgery in these patients promotes inefficient control of heart rate (Kaye, 1977) usually with a high resting HR and a small increase in HR in the first minutes of exercise. Perhaps maximal HR is reached in the recovery period of exercise, and not at peak exercise, taking longer to return to baseline (Guimarães, 1999), as previous shown in Fig. 1.

However, the vasomotor control (neural and hormonal) is not affected by surgery. The changes in this system may appear due to adaptive mechanisms to drug therapy (Toledo, 2002).

Initially it was thought that the denervation was permanent, and there was only the dependence on circulating catecholamines to achieve maximal heart inotropic and chronotropic stimulation (Kaye, 1977). As time passed by and recent studies have been performed, it has been shown that there is a reinnervation process over time after surgery (Fuentes, 2010), because significant higher VO_2, AT (anaerobic threshold), VE (Schwaiblmair, 1999), myocardial function and coronary artery tone are shown after this surgery (Burke, 1995). reinnervation happens in an heterogeneous pattern (Wilson, 1993).

It is known that time after transplantation is recognized as a significant factor correlated to partial autonomic reinnervation among these recipients (Schwaiblmair, 1999). In the majority of recipients with more than one year after cardiac transplantation, cardiac norepinephrine reapers. This support the presence of late heterogeneous sympathetic reinnervation (Wilson, 1993).

Data from Heart Failure Clinics of Heart Institute compare the O_2 consumption increase to the heart rate increase during exercise. It shows that a cardiac transplant recipient at short-term transplantation have the increase of VO_2 during cardiopulmonary exercise test not matched to the increase in HR (Figure 1). The same patient at long-term transplantation showed a closer relationship to this increase (Figure 2), so this might corroborate the idea of partial reinnervation described over time.

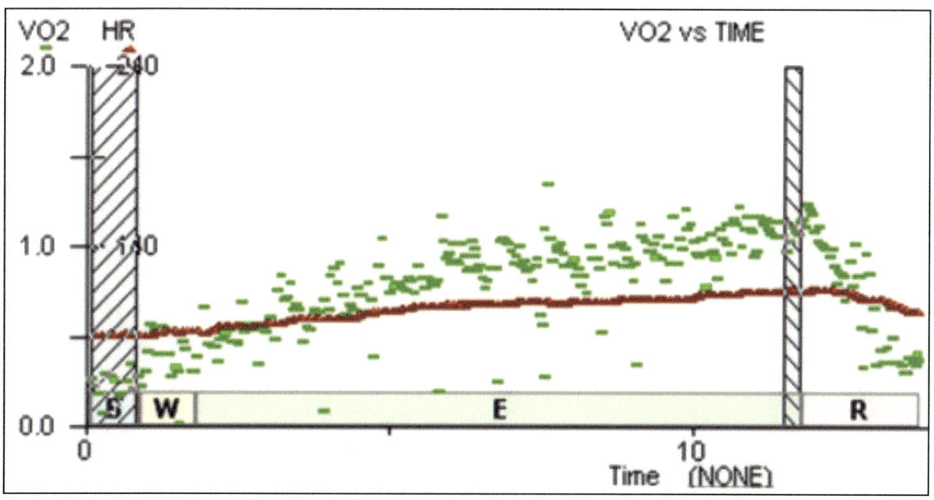

Fig. 1. Response in recent (5 month) post transplant recipients. HR in red, VO_2 in green.

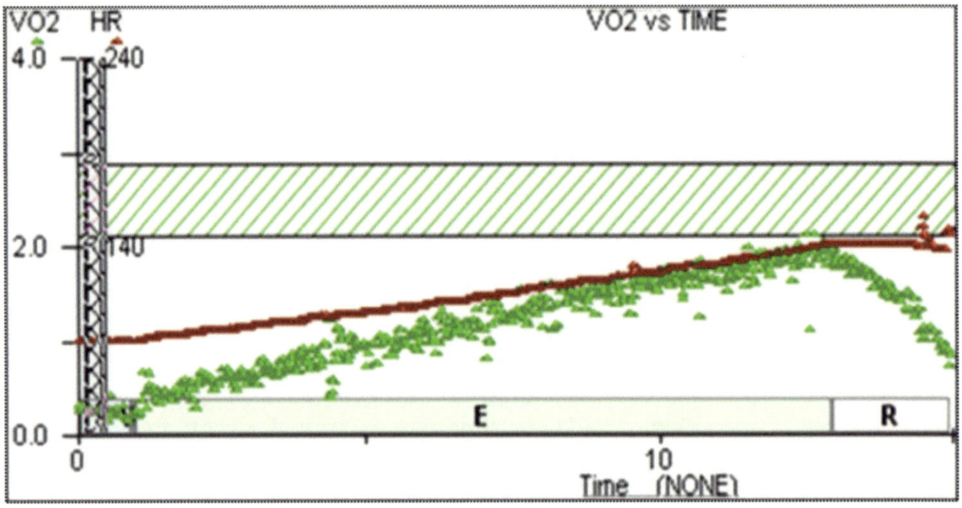

Fig. 2. Response in late (9 year) post transplant recipients. HR in red, VO_2 in green.

Thus, heart rate control acts different from healthy subjects. It becomes more elevated at rest; nevertheless, during exercise, there is gradual delay of its increase from the exercise start to the peak HR. As a result, by the time heart transplant recipients reach their peak HR, it is, indeed, lower than peak HR in healthy subjects. Then, HR decreases in a slow way during the recovery period (Guimarães, 1999). This described finding in exercise could be identified in one of the patient referred to Heart Failure Clinics of Heart Institute, in Brazil (Figure. 3).

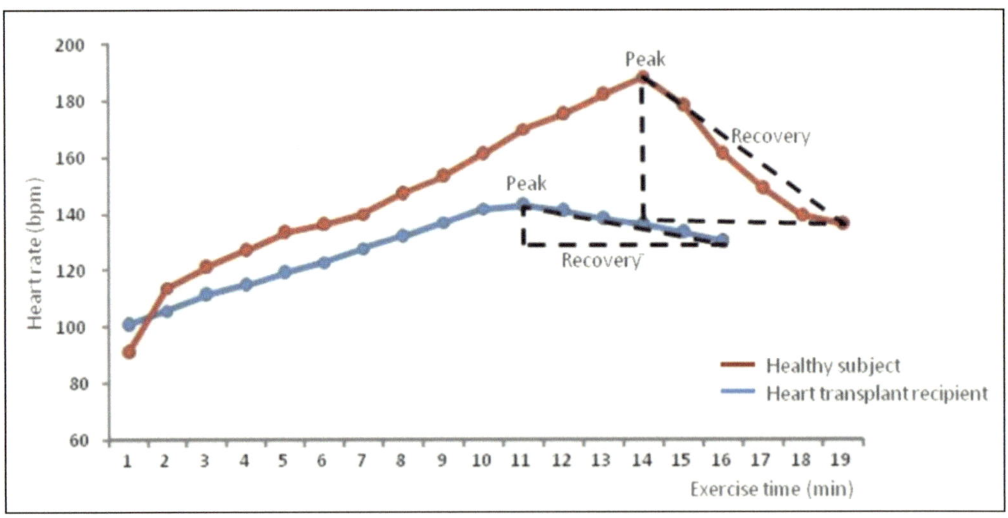

Fig. 3. Heart rate(HR) representation in a sedentary healthy subject (in red) and in a sedentary heart transplantation recipient (in blue).

Comparing the same data from heart transplant recipients and heart failure patients from Heart Failure Clinics of Heart Institute, both, resting HR and peak HR, after surgery becomes significantly higher compared to the same data from healthy subjects, although there is no change in their HR reserve (Figure 4).

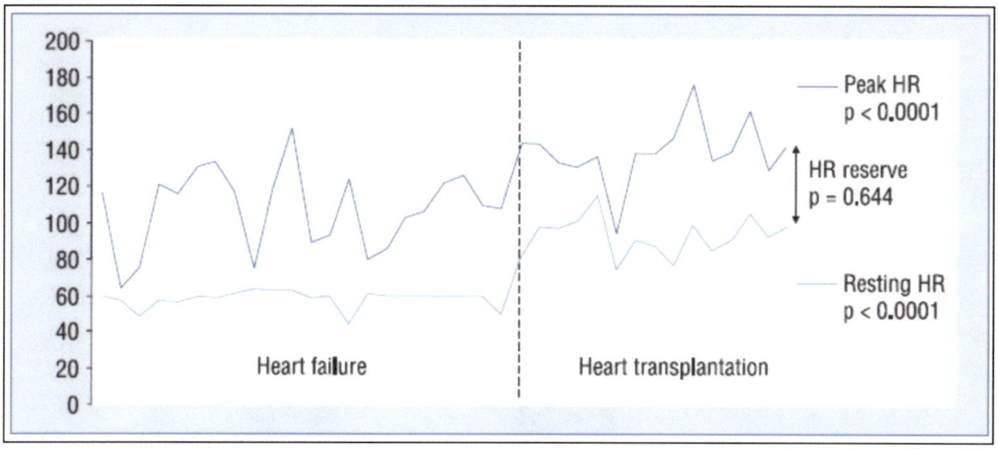

Fig. 4. Resting heart rate, peak heart rate and heart rate reserve in heart failure patients and heart transplant recipients ; HR – heart rate.

Peak heart rate (percentage of the maximum predicted for age) is significant higher in heart transplant recipients than in heart failure patients (Carvalho, 2009a) because the heart remains partially denervated, as it is shown in Figure 5. Thus, the general use of maximum HR adjusted for age recommended by the Task Force, 2006, known as 220 - age, cannot be applied to transplant recipients in order to identify their maximum effort and to prescribe exercise (Casadei, 1992; Guimarães, 2010).

Indeed, no patient reached the maximum heart rate predicted for their age during a treadmill cardiopulmonary exercise test. A heart rate increase in heart transplant patients during cardiopulmonary exercise test comes around 80% of the maximum age-adjusted value (Carvalho, 2009a).

Masked mechanisms responsible for the increase of cardiac output in these patients have close correlation to reaching their physical capacity (Casadei, 1992). In fact, heart transplant recipient's norepinephrine plasma level is lower, at rest, than either healthy or heart failure subjects. But it becomes twice higher than healthy subjects do, after the 6-minute walking test (Guimarães, 2010).

Increases in heart rate and stroke volume at exercise are first linked to the augmented venous return, and later to the increased plasmatic noradrenaline level. Hence, reduced cardiac output response to exercise results in early anaerobic metabolism, acidosis, hyperventilation and diminished physical capacity.

Peak oxygen consumption is reduced in transplant recipients compared to healthy subjects, which may be related to the existence of remaining systolic and diastolic dysfunction (Patel, 2003), muscular atrophy and hormonal abnormalities due to heart failure persistence after transplantation (Gryglewski, 2001), in addition to the use immunosuppressive drugs that reduce exercise capacity, and sympathetic stimulation (Banner, 1989).

A strong relationship was found between percentage of heart rate reserve (%HRR) and percentage of oxygen consumption reserve (%VO_2R) in heart transplant during cardiopulmonary exercise test, as it follows in Figure 6 ($r=0.95$, $p<0.0001$). The %HRR-%VO_2R linear regression between 0 intercept and 1 intercept between the slope of each

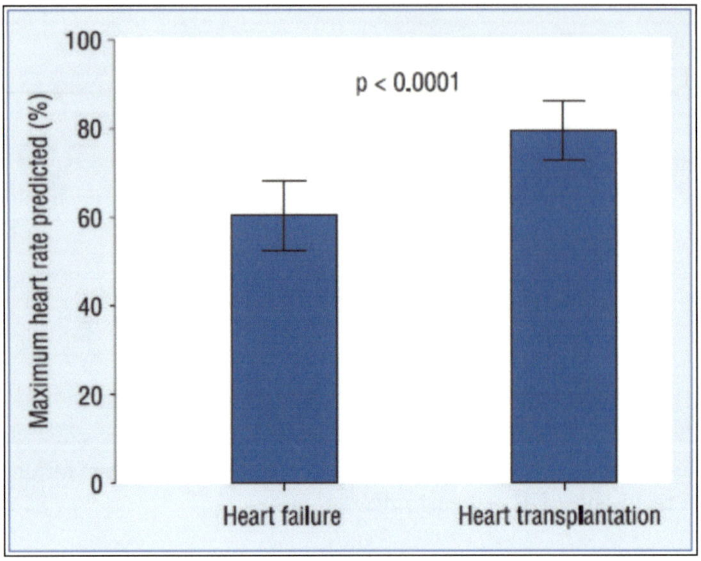

Fig. 5. Mean peak heart rate (percentage of the maximum heart rate predicted for age) in heart failure patients and in heart transplantation recipients. Data is presented as the mean ± 95% confidence interval.

patient showed a slope of −0.23, which means that it is far from the perfection expressed by a slope of 1. Perhaps different terms of heart transplantation and, consequently, different reinnervation status patients could have influenced the imperfect reliability of the %HRR versus %VO_2R (Carvalho, 2009b).

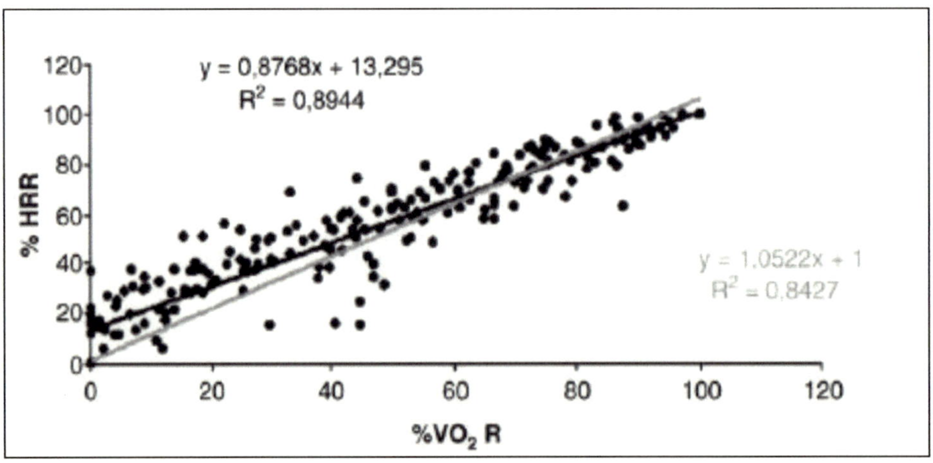

Fig. 6. Percentage of heart rate reserve (%HRR) and percentage of oxygen consumption reserve (%VO_2R)

A close relationship was also found between %peak heart rate versus %peakVO2 (r=0.91, p<0.0001) and absolute heart rate versus absolute VO_2 (r=0.67, p<0.0001). They are expressed in both, Figure 7 and Figure 8, data extracted from Heart Failure Clinics of Heart Institute (Carvalho, 2009b).

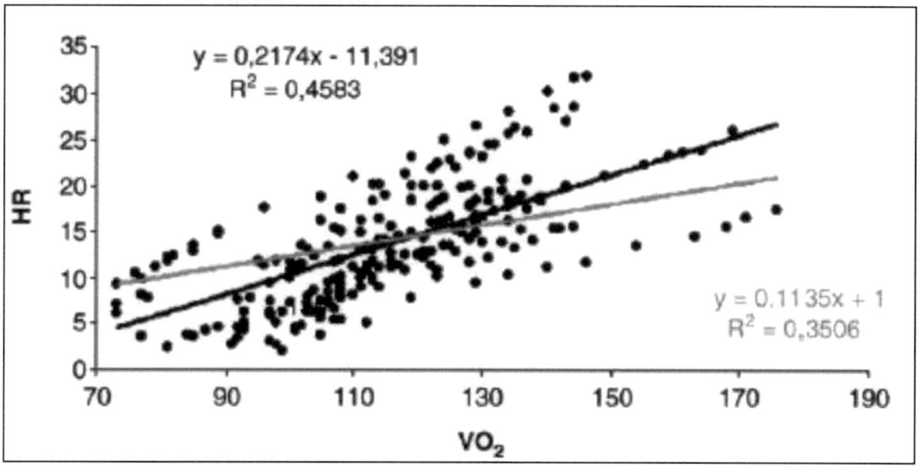

Fig. 7. Heart rate (HR) and peak oxygen consumption (VO_2)

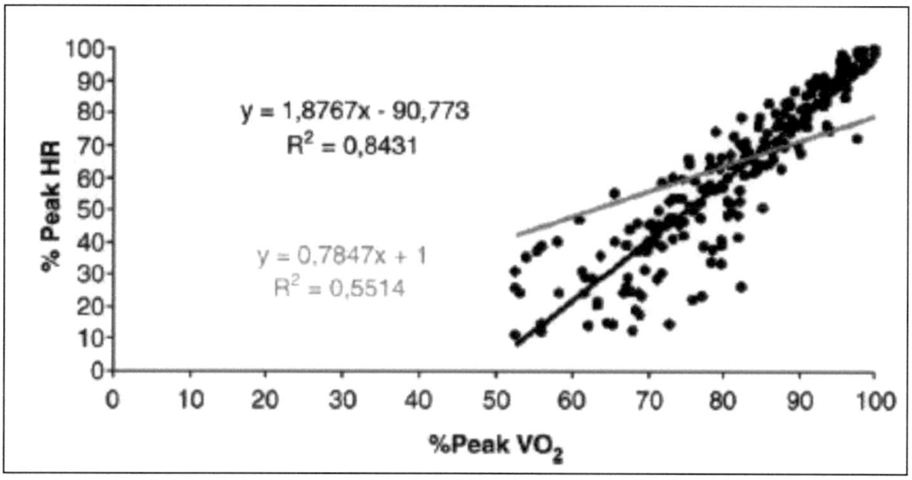

Fig. 8. The plot represents stage by stage regression of the cardiopulmonary exercise test. The grey is the identity line and the black line is regression line. Linear regression between 0 intercept and 1 intercept to percentage of heart rate reserve (%HRR) and percentage of oxygen consumption reserve (%VO_2R) of each patient.

The increased of muscle work and/or activation of the neurohormonal system, in order to maintain, reduced or increase blood pressure and heart rate as an answer to exercise is mainly responsible for the decrease in physical capacity among heart transplant recipients. This decrease in physical capacity after transplantation leads to insufficient production of nitric oxide (Fischer, 2005) and prostacyclin (Guimaraes, 2007), as well as hyperemia dysfunctional, and activation of other compensatory mechanisms. This occurs mainly when there is increased muscle work and/or activation of the neurohormonal system, in order to perform maintenance, reduced or increased blood pressure and heart rate in response to exercise intensity (Poston, 1999; Carvalho, 2009c).

It has also been reported that physical work capacity in heart transplant recipients decrease typically 40% of age-predicted normal levels (Goodman, 2007).

Finally, the reduction in arterial compliance observed after transplant may be due to changes on endothelial dysfunction or vascular mechanisms. Moreover, greater sympathetic nerve activity can lead to increased smooth muscle tone of arteries and, consequently, increase of the vessels stiffness (Taylor, 2003; Degertekin, 2002).

4. Exercise program in heart transplanted patients

Regular physical activity has played important role in the improvement of quality, as demonstrated in studies because regular physical activity may revert or diminish the physiological alterations in transplanted patients (Fig.9) (Guimarães, 2004).

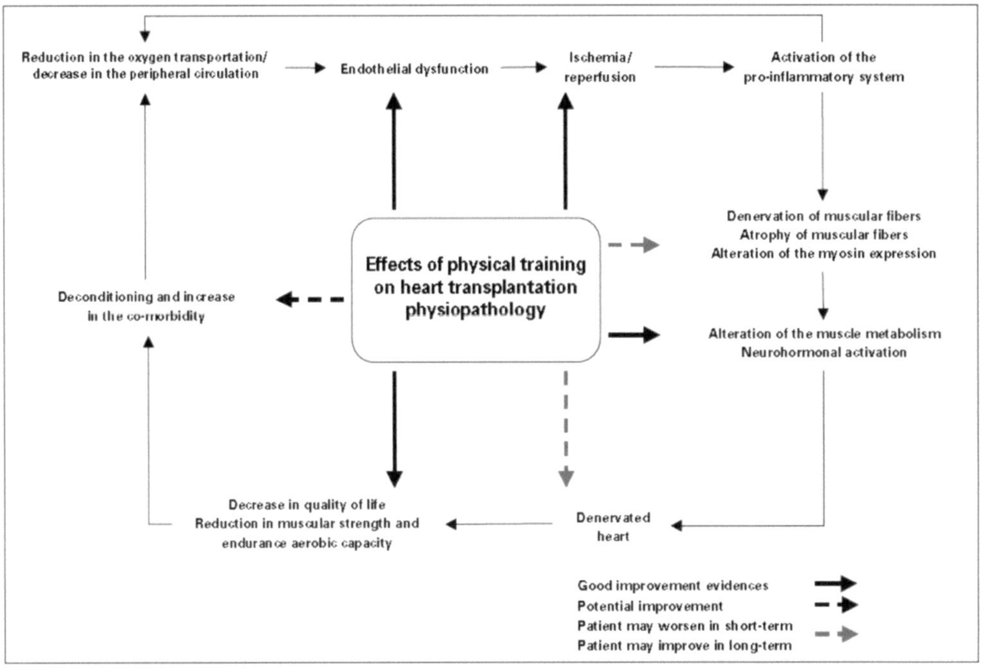

Fig. 9. Association between physical capacity and heart transplantation and the potential role of physical training on the systemic improvement, on the physiopathological effect, on quality of life and on functional capacity

5. Exercise in ICU (intensive care unit)

Even in the earliest days after surgery, the physical therapist will begin to work. Exercise in this scenario is important for several reasons. It aims to restore pulmonary capacity once a median sternotomy procedure is performed and can cause diaphragm reflex inhibition, pain whenever breathing. It also looks for reducing chances of getting lung infections, thromboembolism, bedsores and decrements in peak oxygen consumption (VO_2peak) and related cardiovascular parameters (which may regress approximately 26% within the first 1 to 3 weeks of sustained bed rest) (Braith, 2000) .

Types of exercise include respiratory ones, either with or without equipments, exercises in bed, changing positions in bed, sitting, standing and walking.

Recipients remain in hospital post-transplant depending on their general improvement and lack of complication. Different from pretransplantation hospitalization, which may be prolonged for inotropic support or a ventricular assist device, they leave hospitals soon after surgery because of the risk of infection in a hospital (usually after 2 weeks if there aren't any complications) and are discharged from the unit to a rehabilitation program.

6. Exercise prescription

After heart transplantation patients show physical deconditioning, muscular atrophy, weakness and lower maximal aerobic capacity so regular aerobic/strength training have been studied in both post-heart transplant recipients adults (Keteyian, 1991) and children (Patel, 2008) to study whether it would improve exercise performance. Most programs currently treating orthotopic transplant patients usually provide 6-12 week of exercise training.

In general overview, exercise program improves maximal O2 consumption and, by improving peak heart rate and also improves O_2 delivery in adults after a 10-week exercise program (Keteyian, 1991).

Benefits have also been found in children. After an exercise intervention consisted of aerobic exercise (either running or bicycling for 30 minutes three days/week), plus strength training was performed with elastic bands to specifically exercise biceps and triceps groups for 15-20 min/session was responsible for pediatric heart recipients improvement in their endurance time, peak oxygen consumption and strength.

Studies on aerobic training after cardiac transplantation have distinct characteristics of intensity, type, duration and frequency, so that the evaluation of the results on the effects on the cardiovascular system should be interpreted carefully. Moreover, the intensity of the exercise may enable or help to depress the immune system by hormonal, metabolic and mechanical mechanisms; however, there are no studies about the effect of intensity on the immune response in this population. (Guimarães, 1999).

Knowing the exercise stress tests is necessary information in order to develop a correct exercise prescription. Naughton protocol is more recommended for these patients. Among the parameters, heart rate reflects the cardiac stress, and the rest and maximum, or the metabolic thresholds are used to prescribe the range of exercise intensity and monitor physical training (initially 70% heart rate reserve). (Carvalho, 2009a; Braith, 2000).

Blood pressure during exercise reflects a combination of increased cardiac output and reduced peripheral resistance, thus it should also be considered when prescribing exercise and monitoring it. These hemodynamic variables must be observed during the rehabilitation program for either progression or discontinuation, if necessary.

7. Physical exercise after hospital discharge

Nine months after the surgery procedure, partial reinnervation shows up, but it, yet, promotes inefficient control of heart rate (Bernardini, 1998). This reinnervation can be partially restored over the years. Although heart rate increases after an exercise program (Schwaiblmair, 1999), it remains attenuated, thus, not worth to precise monitor cardiovascular and aerobic exercise prescription. Around 80% of the maximum age-adjusted value could be considered an effort near the maximum, so, it may be a parameter for prescribing exercise (Carvalho, 2009a).

Another good method to prescribe aerobic exercise training in heart transplant recipients without a cardiopulmonary exercise test with gas analysis is by the ratings of perceived exertion (Carvalho, 2009b). In order to achieve this purpose subjects are encouraged to do exercise between a relatively easy rhythm and a slightly tiring one, between 11 and 13 on the Borg Scale as seen in Table 1. (Guimarães, 2008).

Borg Scale	Self-subject fatigue association
6	
7	Very easy
8	
9	Easy
10	
11	Relatively easy
12	
13	Slightly tiring
14	
15	Tiring
16	
17	Very tiring
18	
19	Exhaustive
20	

Table 1. Borg Scale of subject fatigue.

Comparing heart transplant recipients from our lab at Heart Failure Clinics of Heart Institute before and after an exercise program, a more efficient parasympathetic response can be identified (compare the blue line on Figure 3 to the one in Figure 10). In sedentary people after transplantation exercise recovery is significantly slower than in healthy ones (Figure 1), but it becomes close to normal after exercise (Figure 2). This may be explained by the partial restoring function of the **autonomic nervous system** (ANS), especially of the parasympathetic system because a more efficient stimulation in concern of a reduction in heart rate becomes present.

Specific time exercise program is, yet, not precise in order to restore ANS due to total reinnervation, but current data indicates that combined therapy (drug stimulation of reinnervating sympathetic neurons and exercise) can establish better ANS function after orthotopic heart transplantation (Burke, 1995).

Published studies on heart transplant recipients' rehabilitation have shown better hemodynamic function (Braith, 1998b) with dif\ferent training programs. It is clear that physical activity immediately following heart transplantation and adherence to an

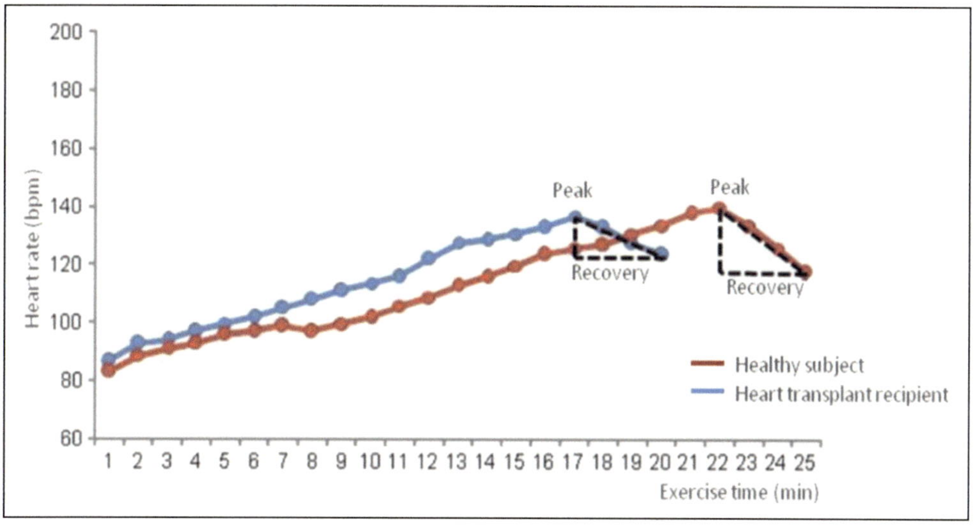

Fig. 10. HR representation after a 12-week exercise program in a healthy subject (in red) and in a heart transplantation recipient (in blue).

individualized program that promotes an active life style helps to restore cardiovascular function (Goodman, 2007). Programs include aerobic exercise, weightlifting, flexibility exercise, or training in both land and water.

Each of the programs has a particularity. Their specifications and attention are concerned to type of exercise, intensity, volume and frequency of the sections. Knowing these differences may help one to better prescribe a training exercise program (Table 2.)

8. Aerobic exercise

Aerobic exercise such as walking, running and cycle ergometer can be prescribed on a continuous or interval kind, depending on experience or protocol used by rehabilitation service. Nonetheless, the intensity of aerobic exercise should be determined according to the workload, if possible at the respiratory compensation point reached during the cardiopulmonary exercise test in combination to exercise at a pace between "relatively easy and slightly tiring", between 11 and 13 on the Borg Scale (Guimarães, 2008). Exercise sessions should be held three times a week with a 5-minute warm up, 30 minutes of aerobic training followed by 5 minutes of recovery and 20 minutes of strength exercises.

9. Weightlifting

Exercise with weights, adjacent to the aerobic exercises, have been recommended after heart transplantation, although hemodynamic function is restored to near normal values, this group of patients still shows a significant decrease in muscle mass and strength, bone rarefaction and histochemical changes in muscle fiber type from type I to type II (Braith, 1998; Lindenfeld, 2004a, Lindenfeld, 2004b).

These persistent changes in the transplant can be minimized with regular practice of resistance training with weights and moderate intensity that must be performed in small

Specification	Aerobic	Weightlifting		Flexibility	Water
		Static	Dynamic		
Type	Interval and continuous training	Main muscle groups	8 to 10 (main muscle groups)	Main muscle groups	Walking (in hot water at 30 or 31°C)
Intensity[ŧ]	60% to 70% peak VO_2 HR between AT and RCP	30 to 75%MVC	40% to 80% 1MR	light to moderate	60% to 70% peak VO_2 HR between AT and RCP
Volume[ŧ]	30 to 40 min	1 to 10 x 6 s	1 x 4 to 6 (avoiding fatigue)	3 a 5 repetitions	30 a 40 min
Frequency	5 x a week	2 x a week^{-1} (5 – 10 x a day)[§]	2 x a week (maximal)	5 x a week	2 x a week
Progression	Respect the Borg scale perception between 13 and 15	Tolerable ROM (initial); Perform contraction under different ROM whenever pain and inflammation get lower. Add load when strength is increased	5-10%-load (a week) ·	In order to stretch soft tissue and either to keep or increase ROM	Respect the Borg scale between 13 and 15
Attention	BP lowering during exercise sections whenever Borg scale perception is greater than previous sections.	Contraction > 10 s may increase BP	-	Respect morphologic al limits in order not to cause injuries.	BP lowering during exercise sections whenever Borg scale perception is greater than previous sections.

Table 2. Practical recommendations for exercise prescription. MVC: maximal voluntary contraction; AT: anaerobic threshold; RCP: respiratory compensation point; 1MR: one maximal repetition test; ROM: range of motion; BP: blood pressure; [ŧ] Subjects were encouraged to begin under their low threshold and increase intensity up to their highest threshold, progressively, as tolerated. [ŧ] Static: 1) from a 6-second contraction at first, to an 8 or 10-second contraction, 2) wait 20-second intermission between contractions; Dynamic: one series of 4 or 6 repetitions without any muscle fatigue; [§]subjects should go from exercising twice a day to 5-10 times a day.

series, with a maximum of ten repetitions for flexors and extensors groups of the upper and lower limbs. This results in reduction of osteoporosis and skeletal muscle myopathies (caused by the use of glucocorticoids), and contributes to the gain in muscle strength and increase in VO_2 peak, at the same time (Lindenfeld, 2004b).

10. Flexibility exercises

Stretching exercises should be conducted to promote gains on range of motion, balance, to stretch the muscles of the neck, lower back, upper and lower limbs. Exercise with elastic can be performed in small series of ten repetitions for each muscle prioritizing posterior trunk and involving large joints of hip, knee, elbow and shoulder.

11. Aquatic exercise

Physical activity in aquatic environment is little reported after cardiac transplantation. However, a case report demonstrated potential benefits of training in heated swimming pool at 30-31°C, 1.40 meters of depth, with sessions of 40 minutes of exercise: 5-minute warm up, 15 minutes of walking on water, 15-minute workout with weights involving large joints and 5 minutes of relaxation. Physical activity in aquatic environment is a well established method of rehabilitation for patients with significant functional limitations and has proven to be effective in cases of obesity after transplantation.

12. Implication of drug therapy in exercise

During the last 25 years there has been a significant increase in survival of patients undergoing heart transplantation (Guba, 2002), generally, as a result of advanced immunosuppressive therapy to control organ rejection since the transplanted heart originates from another organism, and the recipient's immune system attempt to reject it.

But the most widely used therapy is the combination of several drugs that have different modes of action and potential. Some side effects of the use of immunosuppressive medication may appear early in the drug treatment and can be minimized with appropriate modifications and adjustments of schedules and doses (Chart 1, 2 and 3).

Since the late onset side effects must be controlled with the inclusion of specific drugs to control the clinical signs and symptoms of the patient. The latter is represented by corticosteroids, calcineurin inhibitors and TOR inhibitors.

Corticosteroids (Prednisone) act as a nonspecific anti-inflammatory, so the rejection process suffers a direct influence of the recruitment and activation of T-helper lymphocytes. The TOR inhibitors: Tacrolimus (also known as FK-506 or Fujimycin) has a similar action to cyclosporine and is used as a second option to cyclosporine, and Sirolimus, also known as rapamycin, has an inhibitory effect on activation and proliferation of T cells. So, these immunosupressive drugs reduce the infection risk, but may have some undesirable adverse effects (Bortolotto, 1997; Fiorelli, 1996), such as nephrotoxic effects, artery damage and narrowing, left ventricle hypertrophy, increased likelihood of bone fractures and infections. These entire side effects contribute to related health problems over time, so it makes professional responsible for their physical rehabilitation more attempted to effects during exercise as increased blood pressure, transient ischemic attack (TIA).

Moreover, there has been growing clinical consensus that specific training regimens (endurance and resistance) in heart transplant recipients can be efficacious adjunctive therapies in the prevention of immunosuppression-induced side effects and may be an effective countermeasure for corticosteroid-induced osteoporosis and skeletal muscle myopathy.

Heart transplanted recipients who participate in specific resistance training programs successfully restore bone mineral density (BMD) in both the axial and appendicular skeleton to pretransplantation levels, increase lean mass to levels greater than pretransplantation, and reduce body fat. In contrast, those who do not participate in resistance training lose approximately 15% BMD from the lumbar spine early in the postoperative period and experience further gradual reductions in BMD and muscle mass late after transplantation. (Braith, 2000)

Medicine	**Side Effects**	**Exercise limitations**
Corticosteroids (Prednisone)	Hypertention	Left ventricle hypertrophy, damage to the arteries, brain, heart, kidney and even sudden death.
	Hyperglycemia	Damage to the arteries, brain, heart, and kidney.
	Hyperlipidemia	Damage to the arteries, brain, heart, and kidney.
	Diabetes	Damage to the arteries, brain, heart, and kidney, peripheral neuropathy, loss of balance and falls.
	Weight gain	Gallstones and Diabetes.
	Osteoporosis	Bone fracture
	Cushingoid appearance	NA
	Mood changes	Not adherence to an exercise protocol
	Cataract	Incoordination and loss of balance
Calcineurin inhibitors (Cyclosporine)	Kidney vasoconstriction	Nephrotoxicity and sodium retention (which contribute to body plasma volume)
	Hyperkalemia	Cardiopulmonary arrest
	Hypertension	Left ventricle hypertrophy, damage to the arteries, brain, heart, kidney and even death.
	Venous thrombosis	Pulmonary thromboembolism
	Migraine	Not adherence to an exercise protocol
	Tremor	Incoordination
	Paresthesia	Loss of balance and falls
	Gout	Pain and ROM limitation
	Gum hyperplasia	NA
	Hepatotoxicity	NA

Chart 1. Side effects and mainly corticosteroids and calcineurin inhibitor interferences. NA: not applicable. ROM: range of motion.

Medicine	Side Effects	Exercise limitations
Tacrolimus	Kidney vasoconstriction	Nephrotoxicity (similar to cyclosporine)
	Hypertension*	Left ventricle hypertrophy, damage to the arteries, brain, heart, kidney and even sudden death.
	Hyperlipidemia*	Damage to the arteries, brain, heart, and kidney.
	Diabetes #	Damage to the arteries, brain, heart, and kidney, peripheral neuropathy, loss of balance and falls.
Sirolimus	Bone marrow aplasia	Thrombocytopenia, anemia and leukopenia
	Hyperlipidemia	Damage to the arteries, brain, heart, and kidney.
	Peripheral edema	Difficulty on progressing ROM, loss of balance and falls.
	Wound healing impairment.	Incapacity of moving the affected area, not adherence to an exercise protocol.

Chart 2. Side effects and mainly TOR inhibitors interferences. * fewer than cyclosporine's side-effect; # greater than cyclosporine's side-effect;

Medicine	Side Effects	Exercise limitations
Azathioprine	Neutropenia and thrombocytopenia	Increased risk of infections, venous thrombosis, pulmonary thromboembolism anemia, and bleeding.
	Nausea, vomit	Not adherence to an exercise protocol
	Pancreatitis, hepatotoxicity and cancer.	NA
Mycophenolate	Neutropenia	Increased risk of infections
	Nausea, vomit	Not adherence to an exercise protocol

Chart 3. Side effects and mainly antiproliferative agents interferences.

13. Final comments

Heart transplantation is indicated as therapy for patients in the end stage of heart failure. These patients, despite the fact they trade their damaged hearts for functional ones, they remain with several impairments, as muscle weakness, and develop some other disabilities because of the transplantation procedure itself and due to the use of required drugs to control rejection.

Regular physical activity in general has shown potential benefits for the control and reduction of chronic degenerative diseases, which should be incorporated as a therapeutic agent after cardiac transplantation. However, studies on cardiac rehabilitation in transplanted patients are isolated and inconclusive regarding the answer in the long term effect on the immune system, neurohormonal, musculoskeletal and adherence to the program. Furthermore, these studies refer only to cardiovascular training, leaving aside structural and postural changes, such as rotations, shoulder girdle and pelvic misalignments-scapular of the patient, which can be found in the majority who have some functional deviation as stiffed vertebral joints and shorten muscle. Another important aspect that we consider is the socio-cultural reference of transplant patients, which can often limit or even refuse to participate on a physical training program.

The effect of physical conditioning after transplantation is mainly attributed to higher peripheral efficiency, but there has also been found a degree of cardiac adaptation.

In current practice of heart transplant recipients' therapy, further studies are needed to elucidate the role of physical activity on the interaction of physiological and clinical responses in this group of patients.

14. Acknowledgment

Lucas N Pascoalino was supported by Coordination for the Improvement of Higher Level - or Education- Personnel (CAPES)

Guilherme V Guimaraes was supported by Conselho Nacional de Pesquisa (CNPq # 304733/2008-3).

Wish to thank the Agency of the São Paulo Research Foundation (FAPESP # 2007/05639-9)

15. References

Banner NR, Khaghani A, Fitzgerald M, Mitchell AG, Radley-Smith R, Yacoub M. (1989). The expanding role of cardiac transplantation. In: Unger F, ed. Assisted circulation III. Berlin: Springer Verlag. 448-67.

Bernardi L, Valenti C, Wdowczyck-Szulc J, Frey AW, Rinaldi M, Spadacini G, Passino C, Martinelli L, Viganò M, Finardi G. . (1998). Influence of Type of Surgery on the Occurrence of Parasympathetic Reinnervation After Cardiac Transplantation. *Circulation.* 97:1368-74.

Bocchi EA. (1999). Introdução. Diretrizes da Sociedade Brasileira de Cardiologia para Transplante Cardíaco. Arq Bras Cardiol. 73(supl V):5.

Bocchi EA, Fiorelli A. (2001). The Brazilian experience with heart transplantation: a multicenter report. J Heart Lung Transplant. 20(6):637-45.

Bortolotto LA, Silva HB, Bocchi ES, Bellotti G, Stolf N, Jatene AD. (1997). Evolução a Longo Prazo e Complicações da Hipertensão Arterial após Transplante CardíacoArq Bras Cardiol. 69 (5):317-21.

Braith RW, Welsch MA, Mills RM Jr, Keller JW, Pollock ML. (1998) Resistance exercise prevents glucocorticoid-induced myopathy in heart transplant recipients. Med Sci Sports Exerc. 30: 483-9.

Braith RW, Mills RM Jr, Wilcox CS, Davis GL, Wood CE. (1996). Breakdown of blood pressure and body fluid homeostasis in heart transplant recipients. J Am Coll Cardiol. 27: 375-83.

Braith RW, Edwards DG. (2000). Exercise following heart transplantation. Sports Med. 30(3):171-92.

Burke MN, McGinn AL, Homans DC, Christensen BV, Kubo SH, Wilson RF. (1995). Evidence for functional sympathetic reinnervation of left ventricle and coronary arteries after orthotopic cardiac transplantation in humans. Circulation. 91:72-8.

Carvalho VO, Bocchi EA, Pascoalino LN, Guimarães GV. (2009). The relationship between heart rate and oxygen consumption in heart transplant recipients during a cardiopulmonary exercise test. Int J Cardiol. 141(1):158-60.

Carvalho VO, Ruiz MA, Bocchi EA, Carvalho VO, Guimarães GV. (2009). Correlation between CD34+ and exercise capacity, functional class, quality of life and norepinephrine in heart failure patients. Cardiol J. 16(5):426-431.

Carvalho VO, Bocchi EA, Guimarães GV. (2009). The Borg scale as an important tool of self-monitoring and self-regulation of exercise prescription in heart failure patients during hydrotherapy: a randomized blinded controlled trial. Circ J. 73 (10): 1871-6.

Casadei B, Meyer TE, Coats AJ, Conway J, Sleight P. (1992). Baroreflex control of stroke volume in man: an effect mediated by the vagus. *J Physiol.* 448:539–50.

Degertekin M, Serruys PW, Foley DP, Tanabe K, Regar E, Vos J, Smits PC, van der Giessen WJ, van den Brand M, Feyter P, Popma JJ. (2002). Persistent Inhibition of Neointimal Hyperplasia After Sirolimus-Eluting Stent Implantation. Circulation. 106:1610 -3.

Di Rienzo M, Parati G, Castiglioni P, Tordi R, Mancia G, and Pedotti A. (2001). Baroreflex effectiveness index: an additional measure of baroreflex control of heart rate in daily life. Am J Physiol Regulatory Integrative Comp Physiol. 280: R744–51.

Doering LV, Dracup K, Moser DK, Czer LS, and Peter CT. (1996). Hemodynamic adaptation to orthostatic stress after orthotopic heart transplantation. Heart Lung. 25: 339–51.

el-Gamel A, Doran H, Aziz T, Rahman A, Deiraniya A, Campbell C, Yonan NNA. (1998). Natural history and the clinical importance of early and late grade 2 cellular rejection following cardiac transplantation. *Transplant Proc.*30(4):1143-6.

Fiorelli AI, Stolf NAG. (1996). Cuidados no pós-operatório do transplante cardíaco. Rev. Bras. Cir. Cardiovasc., 11(1): 30-8.

Fischer D, Rossa S, Landmesser U. (2005). Endothelial dysfunctional patients with chronic heart failure is independently associated with increased incidence of hospitalization, cardiotransplantation, or death . Eur. Heart J. 26: 65-69.

Fuentes FB, Dolz LM, Bonet LA, Lázaro IS, Manchón JN, Gómez JMS, Raso R, Llin JA, Carranza MJST, Sanz AS. (2010). Normalization of the Heart Rate Response to Exercise 6 Months After Cardiac Transplantation Proceedings. 42: 3186–8.

Kaye MP. (1993). The registry of the International Society for Heart and Lung Transplantation: Tenth official report. J Heart Lung Transplant. 12: 541-8.

Kaye MP, Randall WC, Hageman GR, Geis WP, Priola DV. (1977). Chronology and mode of reinnervation of the surgically denervated canine heart: functional and chemical correlates. Am J Physiol. 233: H431-437.

Keteyian S, Shepard R, Ehrman J, Fedel F, Glick C, Rhoads K, Levine TB. (1991) Cardiovascular responses of heart transplant patients to exercise training. J Appl Physiol. 70(6):2627-31.

Goodman WF, Pitetti KH, Patterson J, Farhoud H. (2007). Exercise capacity following heart transplant: case report on the physical work capacity of a 37 year old competitive cyclist following orthotopic heart transplant. Proceedings of the 3rd Annual GRASP Symposium. Wichita State University. 127-128.

Guba M, von Breitenbuch P, Steinbauer M. (2002) Rapamycin inhibits primary and metastatic tumor growth by antiangiogenesis: Involvement of vascular endothelial growth factor. *Nat Med.* 8: 128–35.

Guimarães GV, Carvalho VO, Bocchi EA. (2008). Reproducibility of the self-controlled Six-minute walking test in heart failure Patients. Clinics. 63(2):201-6.

Guimarães GV, Bacal F, Bocchi EA. (1999). Reabilitação e condicionamento físico após transplante cardíaco. Rev Bras Med Esporte. 5(4):144-6.

Guimarães GV, d'Avila VM, Chizzola PR, Bacal F, Stolf N, Bocchi EA. (2004) Reabilitação física no transplante de coração. Rev Bras Med Esporte. 10(5):408-11.

Guimaraes GV, d'Avila VM, Pires P, Bacal F, Stolf N, Bocchi E. (2007). Acute effects of a single dose of phosphodiesterase type 5 inhibitor (sildenafil) on systemic arterial blood pressure during exercise and 24-hour ambulatory blood pressure monitoring in heart transplant recipients. Transplant Proc. 39(10):3142-9.

Guimaraes GV, d'Avila VM, Bocchi EA, Carvalho VO. (2010). Norepinephrine remains increased in the six-minute walking test after heart transplantation. Clinics. 65(6):587-91. Gryglewski RJ, Chlopicki S, Uracz W, Marcinkiewicz E. (2001). Significance of endothelial prostacyclin and nitric oxide in peripheral and pulmonary circulation. Med. Sci. Monit. 7(1):1-16.

Haywood, Peter R Rickenbacher, Pedro T Trindade, Lars Gullestad, Joseph P Jiang, John S Schroeder, Randall Vagelos, Philip Oyer, Michael B Fowler (1996). Analysis of deaths in patients awaiting heart transplantation: impact on patient selection criteria. Heart. 75:455-62.

Lindenfeld J, Miller GG, Shakar SF, Zolty R, Lowes BD, Wolfel EE, Mestroni L, Page RL, Kobashigawa J. (2004). Drug Therapy in the Heart Transplant Recipient. Part I: Cardiac Rejection and Immunosuppressive Drugs. Circulation 110;3734-40.

Lindenfeld J, Miller GG, Shakar SF, Zolty R, Lowes BD, Wolfel EE, Mestroni L, Page RL, Kobashigawa J. (2004). Drug Therapy in the Heart Transplant Recipient. Part II: Immunosuppressive Drugs. Circulation. 110;3858-65;

Patel AR, Kuvin JT, DeNofrio D, Kinan D, Sliney KA, Eranki KP. (2003). Peripheral vascular endothelial function correlates with exercise capacity in cardiac transplant recipients. *Am J Cardiol.* 91(7):897–9.

Patel JN, Kavey RE, Pophal SG, Trapp EE, Jellen G, Pahl E. (2008). Improved exercise performance in pediatric heart transplant recipients after home exercise training. Pediatr Transplant. 12(3):336-40.

Poston RS, Billingham M, Hoyt G, Pollard J, Shorthouse R, Shorthouse RE, Robbins RC. (1999). Rapamycin Reverses Chronic Graft Vascular Disease in a Novel Cardiac Allograft Model. Circulation. 100:67–74.

Reemtsma K, Hardy MA, Drusin RE, Smith CR, Rose EA. (1985). Cardiac Transplantation. Changing patterns in evaluation and treatment. Ann. Surg. 202(4):418-23.

Reid CJ, YACOUB MA. (1988). Determinants of left ventricular function one year after cardiac transplantation. Br Heart J.59:397-402.

Schwaiblmair M, von Scheidt W, Uberfuhr P. (1999). Functional significance of cardiac reinervation in heart transplant recipients.J Heart Lung Transplant. 18:838–45.

Task Force of the Italian Working Group on Cardiac Rehabilitation Prevention. (2006). Statement on cardiopulmonary exercise testing in chronic heart failure due to left ventricular dysfunction. Eur J Cardiovasc Prev Rehabil. 13: 150–164.

Taylor DO, Edwards LB, Mohacsi PJ. (2003)The Registry of the International Society for Heart and Lung Transplantation: twentieth official adult heart transplant report. J Heart Lung Transplant. 22:616–24.

Toledo E, Pinhas I, Aravot D, Almog Y, Akselrod S. (2002). Functional restitution of cardiac control in heart transplant patients. Am J Physiol Regulatory Integrative Comp Physiol. 282: R900–8.

Wilson RF, Laxson DD, Christensen BV, McGinn AL, Kubo SH. (1993). Regional differences in Sympathetic reinnervation after human orthotopic cardiac transplantation. Circulation. 88:165-171.

Part 2

Chronic Rejection in Cardiac Transplantation

5

Cardiac Allograft Vasculopathy: An Ongoing Challenge in the Care of Heart Transplant Recipients

Brian Clarke and Kiran Khush
Division of Cardiovascular Medicine, Stanford University, Stanford, California, USA

1. Introduction

Cardiac allograft vasculopathy (CAV) represents the most common cause of late graft failure and limits the long-term success of heart transplantation. It is the most common cause of death, in addition to malignancy, in patients who survive the first year after transplant (Taylor *et al.*, 2006). CAV is a diffuse, accelerated form of coronary artery disease in the transplanted heart. Despite improvements in immunotherapy, the incidence of angiographically detected CAV has not changed appreciably over the past two decades. CAV is associated with a relentless course after heart transplantation and immunological and non-immunological interventions have only partially modified its natural history. Treatment of CAV is limited, highlighting the importance of preventive therapies. Re-transplantation for advanced disease is the only definitive therapy, but is limited to select patients. In this chapter, we will review the epidemiology, natural history, clinical manifestations, screening and diagnostic strategies for CAV while emphasizing current treatment strategies designed to prevent or slow the progression of this disease.

2. Pathology

CAV was first described in 1970 as a diffuse, obliterative, accelerated form of arteriosclerosis (Bieber *et al.*, 1970). Pathologically, CAV is distinctly different from traditional coronary atherosclerosis (Table 1). It is characterized by diffuse, concentric intimal smooth muscle hyperplasia involving the entire circumference and length of the vessel, and deposition of neointima in the major epicardial vessels and microvasculature, which progressively obstructs the affected vessel lumen (Figure 1). CAV is further distinguished microscopically as having intense cellular proliferation, composed mainly of smooth muscle cells and inflammatory infiltrates (monocytes and lymphocytes). Specific populations of lymphocytes co-localized with CAV lesions include recipient CD4+ T cells, thus suggesting a role for major histocompatibility complex (MHC) II antigen recognition and processing in the development of CAV. Populations of macrophages and CD8+ T cells have also been localized in CAV lesions, whereas recipient B-cells are rare.

The endomyocardial biopsy has limited sensitivity in the recognition of vasculopathy because it samples only the smallest of intramyocardial arteries and arterioles, which often do not show histologic features of CAV. Reported histologic changes seen in the small arteries in endomyocardial biopsies include concentric intimal thickening with or without foamy macrophages, subendothelial accumulation of lymphocytes, and perivascular fibrosis (Pardo *et al.,* 1997). Evidence of myocardial ischemia, such as myocytolysis, frank coagulation necrosis, and healing ischemic lesions as well as interstitial, perivascular, and replacement fibrosis can be seen (Neish *et al.,* 1992). Identification of myocardial injury should raise the suspicion of CAV as the cause of graft dysfunction. The absence of these findings, however, does not necessarily rule out the presence of CAV.

3. Pathogenesis

The development of CAV represents a complex interaction between acute and chronic immune activation via an allo-immune pathway and alloantigen-independent non-immune mechanisms that ultimately lead to inflammation and endothelial injury, the precursor to CAV. (Figure 2). Immunologic events appear to be most important, since CAV develops in the donor's coronary arteries but not the recipient's vasculature. The donor coronary artery endothelial cells express major histocompatibility complex (MHC) class I and class II antigens, and thus appear to be primary targets of the cell-mediated and humoral immune responses. These antigens are thought to be recognized by recipient CD8+ and CD4+ T cells and these activated lymphocytes secrete cytokines (interleukins, interferons, and tumor necrosis factors), which promote proliferation and further activation of allo-reactive T cells, monocytes, and macrophages. Macrophages are then recruited to the intima where they elaborate cytokines (IL-1, IL-6, tumor necrosis factor TNF alpha) and growth factors [platelet derived growth factor (PDGF), insulin-like growth factor-I (IGF-I), transforming growth factor-alpha (TGF-alpha), TGF-beta-1], leading to smooth muscle cell proliferation and synthesis of extracellular matrix (Libby P & Tanaka H, 1994).

T cell activation also stimulates the expression of adhesion molecules, [intercellular cell adhesion molecule-1 (ICAM-1), vascular cell adhesion molecule-1 (VCAM-1), P-selectin] thereby "activating" endothelial cells, enabling recruitment of proinflammatory cells from the vasculature and the initiation of the immune response and subsequent development of CAV. (Briscoe *et al.,* 1995)

Pathologic characteristic	CAV	Native CAD
Lesion morphology	Diffuse, concentric (variable)	Focal, proximal, eccentric
Vessels involved	Intramyocardial, epicardial branches	Epicardial, spares intramyocardial branches
Collateral vessels	Minimal	Often extensive
Initial Lesion	Smooth muscle proliferation	Fatty streaks
Internal Elastic Lamina	Intact	Disrupted
Endothelial lymphocytes	Sometimes	Absent
T-cell location	Subendothelial	Edge of plaque

Table 1. Characteristics of cardiac allograft vasculopathy compared to traditional coronary atherosclerosis in the native heart.

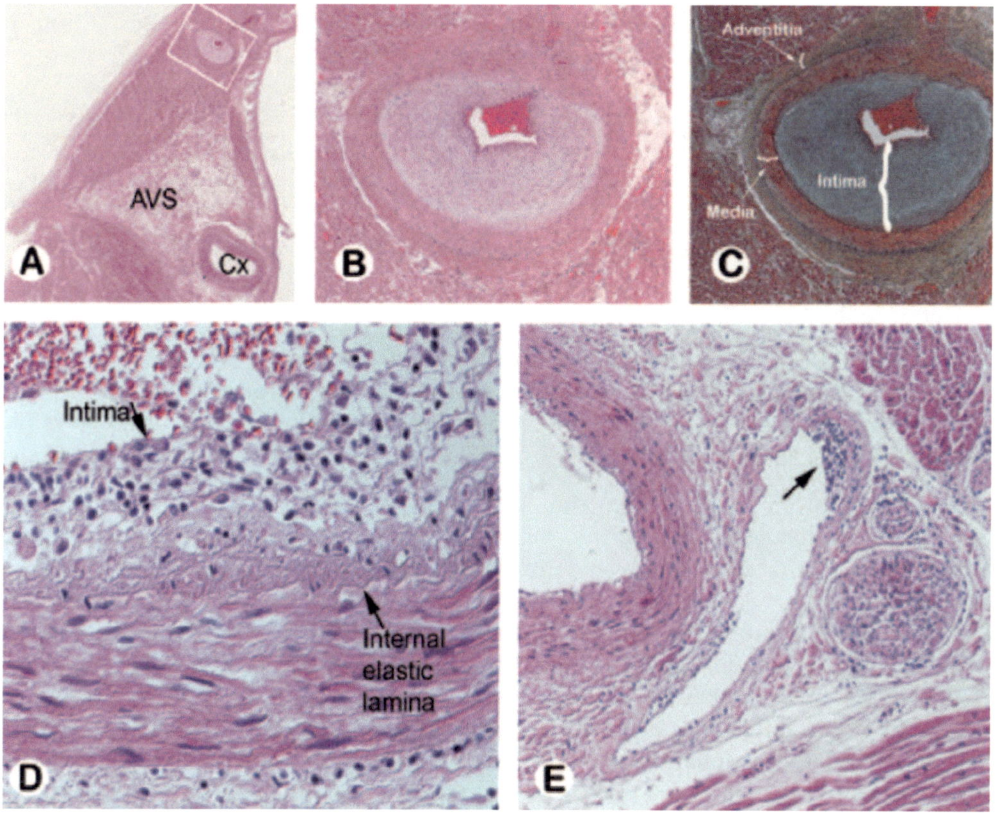

Fig. 1. Cardiac allograft vasculopathy. (A) Photomicrograph of the left atrium and ventricle with the left circumflex (Cx) artery noted at the atrioventricular sulcus (AVS) from a patient who died of CAV 3 years post transplant. (B,C) Intramyocardial branch of circumflex artery (from inset A) supplying the atrium shows marked intimal proliferation with preservation of the elastic lamina and normal medial layer (hematoxylin-eosin (B) and Movat pentachrome (C)). (D,E) Subendothelial lymphocytic infiltration is seen in a small epicardial artery (D) and in an intramyocardial vein (arrow E). Reprinted from Tan CD, Baldwin WM, Rodriguez ER. Update on Cardiac Transplantation Pathology. Arch Pathol Lab Med. 2007;131:1169-1191 with permission from *Archives of Pathology and Laboratory Medicine.* Copyright 2007. College of American Pathologists.

Non -immune mechanisms implicated in the development of CAV include inflammatory injury due to recipient hypertension, dyslipidemia, diabetes and insulin resistance, and obesity, in addition to ischemia-reperfusion injury during organ procurement. Endothelial cell dysfunction resulting from inflammatory injury predisposes to thrombosis, vasoconstriction, and vascular smooth muscle cell proliferation. Reperfusion injury increases expression of endothelin 1, which is associated with post-transplant ischemic fibrosis and subsequent development of arteriopathy, in addition to generating free radicals that promote the expression of such inflammatory adhesion molecules and subsequent leukocyte recruitment (Ferri *et al.*, 2002). More research is needed in the field of organ preservation, possibly targeting specific cellular processes to minimize reperfusion injury. Endothelial injury and dysfunction, regardless of the mechanism, seems to be the key inciting event and the common pathway for the development of CAV.

4. Risk factors

Many risk factors for the development of CAV have been identified and can be broadly divided into donor-specific factors, recipient-specific factors and donor-recipient factors, with the latter being predominantly immune mediated (Table 1).

4.1 Donor factors

Donor factors include a history of hypertension, diabetes, male sex, and history of tobacco use. Older donor hearts confer a higher risk of CAV development compared to younger donor hearts, and this risk appears most significant with donors older than 50 years (Al-Khaldi *et al.*, 2006; Nagji *et al.*, 2010).

Donor mode of death has also been shown to have associations with the development of CAV. Explosive modes of brain death, including gunshot wound to the head, accidental head trauma, or a rapidly progressive intracranial hemorrhage have also been associated with development of CAV after transplantation (Mehra *et al.*, 2004a). It has been demonstrated that rapid brain death induces a calcium overflow injury that affects conduction tissue, coronary artery smooth muscle, and myocardial cells (Cohen *et al.*, 2007; Novitzky *et al.*, 1988). There is also a generalized activation of macrophage-associated cytokines, an up-regulation of immunoregulatory and adhesion cell molecules with subsequent endothelial inflammation and dysfunction, in addition to increased levels of circulating catecholamines, all of which may negatively impact the graft response after heart transplantation (Segel *et al.*, 2002; Takada *et al.*, 1998).

The role of transmitted native vessel atherosclerosis is controversial and conflicting. Studies utilizing serial coronary artery intravascular ultrasound (IVUS) found donor lesions did not significantly change after transplantation (Jimenez *et al.*, 2001). However a maximal intimal thickness ≥ 0.5mm at baseline (1 month post transplant) was one of the strongest predictors of plaque progression at one year in another study (Yamasaki *et al.*, 2011). In another observational study, donor lesions (defined by intimal thickness > 0.5mm by IVUS at 1 month post transplant) did not have a greater increase in intimal thickness compared to other sites without donor lesions, however the incidence of angiographically apparent CAV up to three years after transplant was higher in patients with donor transmitted lesions with no apparent effect on 3 year mortality (Li H *et al.*, 2006).

Hepatitis C infection (HCV) in donor hearts increases recipient mortality with mortality rates in one study of 16.9% at 1 year, 41.8% at 5 years, and 50.6% at 10 years, compared to recipients of hepatitis C negative donors who had 8.2%, 18.5%, and 24.3% mortality, respectively (Gasink *et al.*, 2006). Recipients with HCV-positive donor hearts were more likely to die secondary to CAV. Other studies also note higher rates of CAV in recipients of HCV + donor hearts, possibly related to HCV viremia in a significant proportion of these recipients; the exact mechanism however, is not completely understood (Haji *et al.*, 2004). Hepatitis B seropositivity (HBV) has been correlated with increased rates of CAV. In one observational study, HBV seropositivity, defined as either the donor or recipient being hepatitis B core antibody positive, was associated with higher rates of CAV at 1 year compared to cases where neither the donor nor recipient were HBV seropositive (Haji SA *et al.*, 2006).

4.2 Recipient factors

Recipient factors that are associated with the development of CAV include male sex, pre-transplant ischemic heart disease, and higher body mass index (Costanzo *et al.*, 1998; Taylor *et al.*, 2007). Traditional cardiac risk factors in the recipient including hypertension, diabetes, dyslipidemia and smoking also increase the risk of developing CAV (Sanchez *et al.*, 2008). Importantly, hypertension, dyslipidemia and diabetes are commonly induced post transplant as side effects of immunosuppressant therapy with calcineurin inhibitors and steroids. The prevalence of hypertension increases after transplant from 74.4% at one year to 98.5% at 10 years (Taylor *et al.*, 2007). The incidence of diabetes after heart transplant ranges from 15% to 20% (Martinez-Dolz *et al.*, 2005).

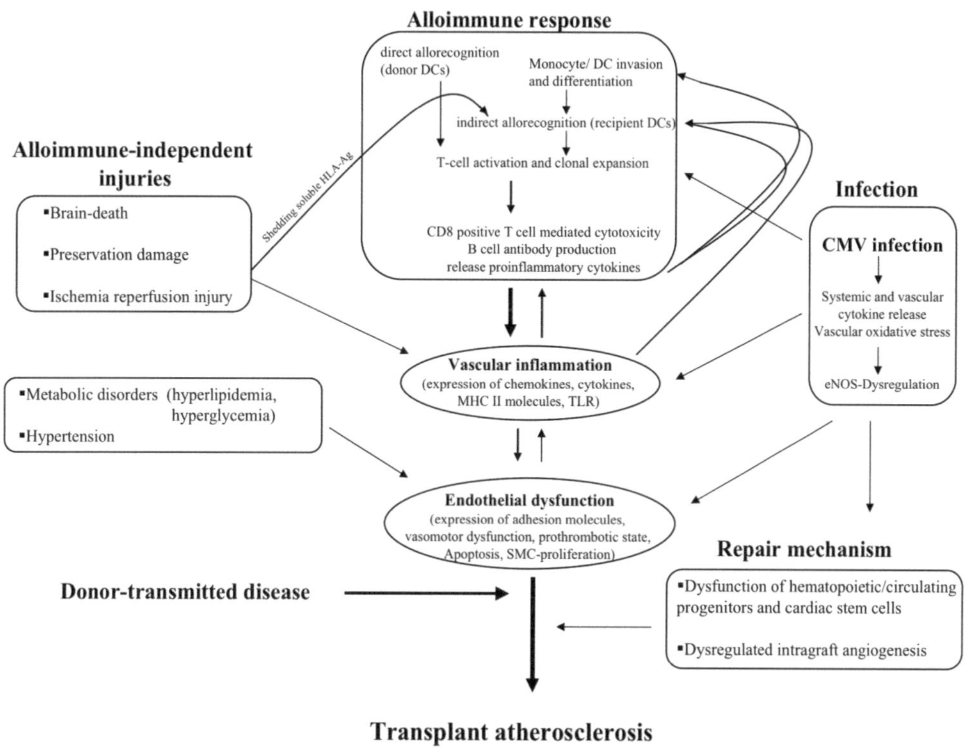

Fig. 2. Pathobiology of Cardiac Allograft Vasculopathy. Reprinted from Schmauss D and Weis M. Cardiac allograft vasculopathy: recent developments. Circulation 2008;117:2131-2141 with permission from Wolters Kluwer Health. Copyright 2008.

4.3 Donor-recipient factors

Donor-recipient factors that increase risk of CAV include episodes of high-grade cellular rejection during the first year after transplantation, HLA-DR mismatches, antibody mediated rejection (including asymptomatic AMR), and cytomegalovirus (CMV) infection.

The total cellular rejection score at six months increases the risk of CAV by almost threefold (Raichlin *et al.*, 2009). The total cellular rejection score is assigned based on ISHLT grading as 0R = 0, 1R = 1, 2R = 2, 3R = 3, and normalized by dividing the cumulative scores for the total number of biopsies taken during the 6 month intervals. Antibody-mediated rejection increases the incidence of CAV by 10% at one year and by 36% at five years (Michaels *et al.*, 2003). Asymptomatic AMR, defined as histologic evidence of AMR, including endothelial swelling, interstitial hemorrhage, interstitial edema and neutrophil infiltration and/or immunoperoxidase staining showing CD-68 positive macrophages within capillary cells and C4d complement coating the walls of the myocardial capillaries, in patients without symptoms or any evidence of graft dysfunction, increases the risk of developing CAV compared to those with no AMR (We *et al.*, 2009).

CMV disease appears to increase the risk of early-onset CAV –an effect that may be mediated via immune mechanisms rather than a direct consequence of the infective organism (Weill *et al.*, 2001). CMV infection in endothelial cells, such as those lining the donor coronary arteries, leads to a local proinflammatory state and subsequent increased production of vascular cell adhesion molecule (VCAM)-1, alterations in cell surface MHC I and II molecules, and an increase in proinflammatory cytokines and growth factors. This causes endothelial cell/smooth muscle cell proliferation and narrowing of the vessel lumen. CMV may also cause endothelial dysfunction leading to CAV by impairing the nitric oxide synthase pathway. (Hosenpud *et al.*, 2003; Koskinen 1993; Van Dorp *et al.*, 1989). Nitric oxide prevents vascular inflammation and lesion formation in the vessel wall by inhibiting platelet and leukocyte adherence and by suppressing vascular smooth muscle cell proliferation. CMV infection of the endothelium increases expression of endothelial surface adhesion molecules and promotes mononuclear adhesion, activation, and transendothelial migration within the vasculature. In addition, CMV is a stimulus of plasma ADMA (asymmetric dimethylarginine) accumulation, the endogenous inhibitor of nitric oxide synthase. (Weis M *et al.*, 2004)

Donor Factors
Age (>50 years), Sex (male) and Mode of Death
History of hypertension, diabetes, smoking
? Donor Transmitted Atherosclerosis
Hepatitis B & C infection
Recipient Factors
Age (>40 years), Sex (male)
Hypertension, dyslipidemia, obesity, smoking
Insulin resistance/Diabetes
Hepatitis B
Donor – Recipient Interaction
Rejection (cellular and antibody mediated)
CMV disease

Table 2. Risk factors for the development of cardiac allograft vasculopathy

5. Clinical manifestations

Early CAV is clinically silent, and ischemia is usually not evident until the disease is far advanced. Patients are most often diagnosed by routine angiographic surveillance or loss of allograft function by surveillance imaging with negative rejection studies. Clinically, patients present with heart failure symptoms and are found to either have new onset systolic or diastolic dysfunction in the absence of acute cellular or antibody mediated rejection, or may present with ventricular arrhythmias and sudden cardiac death. Patients rarely present with chest pain, due to de-innervation of the cardiac allograft at the time of transplantation. However, 25-40% of patients develop some degree of re-innervation post transplant, manifest primarily by return of heart rate response and less often, ischemic chest pain (De Marco *et al.*, 1995).

6. Epidemiology and natural history

CAV is detectable by coronary angiography in approximately 10% of heart transplant recipients within the first year, in 32% - 50% by 5 years, and in an even greater number of recipients when detected by intravascular ultrasound (Pflugfelder *et al.*, 1993). Once mild disease is identified angiographically, the likelihood of progression to severe CAV within 5 years is approximately 19% (Costanzo *et al.*, 1998). Lack of development of CAV at 1 year post-transplant identifies a group who are likely to remain free of clinical events through 6 years of follow up (Luyt *et al.*, 2003). In patients with at least 1 focal stenosis ≥40%, survival was 67% at 1 year, 44% at 2 years, and 17% at 5 years. With 3 vessels involved, survival was 13% at 2 years (Keogl *et al.*, 1992). The overall likelihood of death or re-transplantation as a result of CAV is approximately 50% for severe CAV (Costanzo *et al.* 1998).

Graft function is an important component in evaluating severity of CAV. Patients with CAV and LV dysfunction have significantly lower 5-year survival compared with CAV patients without LV dysfunction (60% vs. 90%) (Stork *et al.*, 2006). Patients with restrictive cardiac physiology [E to A velocity ratio >2, shortened isovolumetric relaxation time (<60msec), shortened deceleration time (≤150ms), or restrictive hemodynamics (right atrial pressure >12mmHg, pulmonary capillary wedge pressure >25mmHg, cardiac index <2.0)] in the presence of preserved LV systolic function and CAV also have a lower 5-year survival than heart transplant patients without restrictive physiology (Itagaki *et al.*, 2007).

7. Diagnosis

Coronary angiography and assessment of cardiac allograft function remains the cornerstone for diagnosis of CAV. Anatomic abnormalities characteristic of CAV include gradual, distal, diffuse, concentric tapering ("distal pruning") of the major epicardial arteries with obliteration of the small branching vessels. Discrete epicardial stenoses are less likely (Figure 3). As early CAV is asymptomatic, routine screening with annual coronary angiography (with or without intravascular ultrasound) is standard practice among the majority of transplant centers in the first 3-5 years post transplant. After this time period, there are different practice patterns for assessment of CAV, depending on individuals' risk factor profile for CAV, graft function, renal function, and clinical status. As CAV is a concentric process, early disease may be overlooked if prior angiograms are not compared. For this reason, baseline angiography is usually performed 4-6 weeks post transplant.

In 2010, the ISHLT working group proposed standardized nomenclature for CAV (Table 3) (Mehra *et al.*, 2010). This system defined CAV as not significant, mild, moderate, and severe based on angiographic appearance. Angiography is a very useful test for detecting lesions

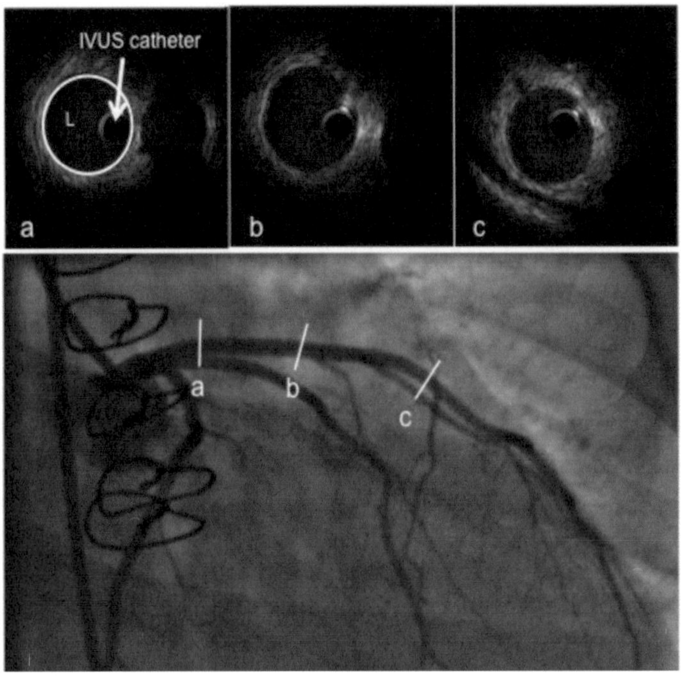

(A)

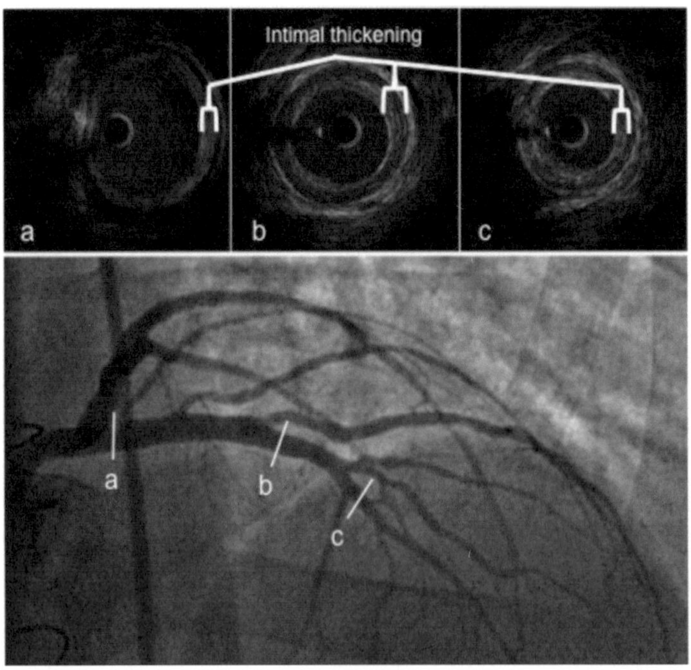

(B)

Fig. 3. Angiography and IVUS imaging demonstrating (A) normal coronary arteries and (B) cardiac allograft vasculopathy. (L= coronary artery lumen).

located in epicardial arteries and the main branches, however the main limitation of angiography is low sensitivity, especially in those mild cases in which an apparently normal examination can underestimate the presence of CAV. This is primarily due the vascular remodeling that occurs early in the disease in which there is no compromise in luminal diameter (Nissen 2001). Repeated angiography is recommended for the follow-up of patients with moderate lesions or for patients with symptoms leading to the suspicion of CAV.

Intra-vascular ultrasound (IVUS) at coronary angiography has been evaluated as an adjunctive modality for assessing and diagnosing early CAV. Angiography depicts only a 2-dimensional silhouette of the lumen whereas IVUS allows a reproducible view of both actual lumen diameter, as well as the appearance and thickness of the intima and media. As the intima begins to thicken, the vessel area enlarges as a compensatory mechanism to preserve luminal area. Therefore, 'angiographically normal' coronary arteries may in fact have significant CAV.

IVUS parameters include intimal thickness, intimal index, and change in maximal intimal thickness at a reference point, total atheroma volume, and percentage of atheroma volume. IVUS can detect occult disease in angiographically normal sites and has emerged as the optimal diagnostic tool for early detection. CAV is considered present when the intimal thickness is >0.3mm (Rickenbacher *et al.*, 1995). The presence of moderate to severe intimal thickening by IVUS is predictive of the future development of angiographically apparent CAV. IVUS-detected maximal intimal thickness (MIT) greater than 0.3mm at 1 year is associated with a 4-year actuarial survival of 73% versus 96% among those with less than 0.3mm of intimal thickening (Rickenbacher *et al.*, 1995). A change in MIT of ≥ 0.5mm at a specific site in the coronary tree within the first year after transplant predicts outcomes at 5 years related to the development of angiographic CAV, mortality and myocardial infarction (Kobashigawa *et al.*, 2005; Tuzcu *et al.*, 2005). Death or graft loss occurred in 21% versus 6%, non-fatal major adverse events or death/graft loss in 46% versus 17% and angiographically apparent disease in 65% versus 33% in those with a change in MIT ≥ 0.5mm between baseline and 1-year (Kobashigawa *et al.*, 2005) versus those with a lesser degree of intimal thickening. With >0.6mm intimal thickening, patients are 10 times more likely to experience a cardiac event and for those who developed cardiac events, 62% of patients had 'normal' angiograms (Mehra *et al.*, 1995).

In patients with stable graft function and no history of CAV, most centers alternate coronary angiography with dobutamine stress echocardiography after 3-5 years; reserving invasive catheterization to every other year. The sensitivity and specificity of dobutamine stress echocardiography compared with coronary angiography and IVUS for detecting CAV is approximately 80% and 88% respectively (Derumeaux *et al.*, 1995; Spes *et al.*, 1999). A normal DSE incorporating M-mode measurement of wall thickening predicts an uneventful clinical course (Spes *et al.*, 1999).

Computed tomographic angiography, although useful in detecting traditional atherosclerosis, has limitations in heart transplant recipients. The major drawbacks with the routine use of 16 or 64 slice multidetector CT in this population include the high heart rate of most heart transplant recipients (due to cardiac vagal denervation) that may compromise imaging quality, contrast-induced nephropathy and radiation. However, compared with

ISHLT CAV_0 (not significant)	No detectable angiographic lesion
ISHLT CAV_1 (Mild)	Angiographic left main (LM) <50%, or primary vessel with maximum lesion of <70%, or any branch stenosis <70% (including diffuse narrowing) without allograft dysfunction
ISHLT CAV_2 (Moderate)	Angiographic LM <50%; a single primary vessel ≥ 70% stenosis, or isolated branch stenosis ≥ 70% in branches of 2 systems, without allograft dysfunction
ISHLT CAV_3 (Severe)	Angiographic LM ≥ 50%, or ≥ 2 primary vessels ≥ 70% stenosis, or isolated branch stenosis ≥70% in all 3 systems; or ISHLT CAV 1 or 2 with allograft dysfunction (defined as LVEF ≤ 45%, usually in the presence of regional wall motion abnormalities) or evidence of significant restrictive physiology (which is common but not specific)

Table 3. The International Society for Heart and Lung Transplantation Recommended Nomenclature for Cardiac Allograft Vasculopathy. 'Primary vessel' denotes the proximal and middle 33% of the LAD, circumflex, ramus and the dominant or co-dominant right coronary artery with the posterior descending and posterolateral branches. 'Secondary branch vessel' includes the distal 33% of the primary vessels or any segment within a large septal perforator, diagonals and OM branches or any portion of a non-dominant RCA. Restrictive physiology is defined as symptomatic heart failure with echocardiographic E to A velocity ratio >2, shortened isovolumetric relaxation time (<60msec), shortened deceleration time (<150msec) or restrictive invasive hemodynamics (right atrial pressure >12mmHg, pulmonary capillary wedge pressure >25mmHg, cardiac index <2L/min/m^2)

IVUS, the sensitivity, specificity, positive and negative predictive values for the detection of CAV by dual source CT were 85%, 84%, 76%, and 91% respectively (Schepis *et al.*, 2009). Magnetic resonance coronary angiography, at present, shows limited sensitivity for detecting CAV and positron emission tomography (PET) has not yet been well studied (Muehling *et al.*, 2003).

Serum biomarkers provide important clues to molecular and structural changes within the transplanted heart. The role of inflammation has been demonstrated by the elaboration of inflammatory cytokines in patients with CAV. Elevated CRP levels have been shown to be associated with increased risk of developing CAV, suggesting a link between systemic and local inflammation within the coronary artery of the transplanted heart (Arora *et al.*, 2010; Raichlin *et al.*, 2007). However, it is not clear if CRP is merely a marker or if it is involved in CAV pathogenesis. Persistently elevated troponin I levels after heart transplantation are associated with an increased risk of development of CAV (Labarrere *et al.*, 2000). Elevated BNP has also been correlated with the development of CAV (Mehra *et al.*, 2004b). BNP may be useful in combination with angiographic findings in predicting outcomes, with 50% of patients with high BNP levels and angiographic CAV experiencing cardiac death (Tsutsui *et al.*, 2001). Biomarkers may hold predictive correlation, but are not used routinely for the evaluation of CAV.

8. Prevention and treatment

Therapeutic options in CAV can be thought of in terms of prevention and treatment. Medical therapy aims to slow, halt, or even reverse the intimal proliferation, concentric luminal loss and arterial obliteration that characterize CAV. Preventive therapy targets traditional cardiac risk factors (diabetes mellitus, hyperlipidemia and hypertension) and aggressive treatment of rejection episodes. Rapidly progressive CAV within the first year after heart transplant strongly predicts all-cause mortality, myocardial infarction, and the subsequent development of angiographically severe CAV. Accordingly, prophylactic strategies must be implicated very early to induce significant improvement in long-term prognosis.

Statins have been associated with reduced progression of CAV, and routine administration of statins to all patients after transplant has clearly reduced the mortality and progression of the disease (Wenke *et al.*, 2003). A meta-analysis based on the published results of three randomized clinical trials determined that the use of statins decreased 1-year mortality following heart transplantation from 17.1% to 5.4% (Mehra *et al.*, 2004c). The introduction of routine anti-CMV drugs to all CMV seropositive patients (donor or recipient or both) for at least 3 months and in some centers up to 6 months has lowered the incidence of CMV infection and its impact on the graft. In a randomized study, patients receiving gancyclovir were significantly more likely to remain free of CAV for 5 years post transplant (Valantine *et al.*, 1999).

There are small studies that suggest calcium channel blockers, such as diltiazem, are effective in slowing the progression of CAV (Schroeder *et al.*, 1993). ACE inhibitors have been associated with plaque regression and improved survival for established CAV , however pre-emptive therapy with ACE inhibitors has unknown preventative effects (Bae *et al.*, 2006). Currently, there is little definitive evidence to suggest that calcium channel blockers or ACE inhibitors are effective in reducing the incidence or slowing the progression of CAV.

Diabetes is common in cardiac transplant recipients and most heart transplant patients are markedly insulin resistant and demonstrate many of the features of compensatory hyperinsulinemia, including the atherogenic and proinflammatory profile of the metabolic syndrome (Potena L & Valantine H, 2007). Patients with high plasma glucose or insulin concentrations after oral glucose intake have greater intimal thickness and are less likely to be free of CAV and have significantly lower survival during 5 years of follow up than patients with low glucose and insulin levels (Valantine *et al.*, 2001). Specific therapies shown to be effective in correcting insulin resistance, such as the thiazolidinediones, offer potential new therapeutic targets for CAV prevention, however the clinical studies are lacking.

Owing to the diffuse nature of vasculopathy, conventional therapeutic approaches including percutaneous coronary intervention and coronary artery bypass grafting are optional only late in the course and are not always successful or even feasible.

Immunosuppression continues to represent the principal means of pharmacologic prophylaxis against and treatment of allograft vasculopathy, with the development and introduction of the proliferation signal inhibitors (PSI) sirolimus and everolimus representing the greatest advance achieved to-date in this field. PSI's are powerful immunosuppressant drugs that inhibit cellular proliferation and have shown the ability to reduce, and even reverse, coronary intimal growth in established CAV and reduce the incidence of CAV in *de novo* transplant patients through a variety of mechanisms, including a reduction in CMV infection and decreased rejection episodes. (Eisen *et al.*, 2003; Keogh *et al.*, 2004).

In a prospective multi-center randomized double blind control trial, patients who received everolimus, cyclosporine and steroids versus azathioprine, cyclosporine and steroids had a significant reduction in the incidence of CAV at 12 months (35.7% versus 52.8%), fewer grade ≥ 3A cellular rejections (21.3% versus 30.6%) and CMV infection (12% versus 41.4%) (Eisen *et al.*, 2003). Similar results were found with sirolimus (Keogh *et al.*, 2004). The long-term results of both studies demonstrate a trend toward a lower incidence of severe vasculopathy in the group that is maintained on PSI with patients treated with everolimus having significantly lower rates of major cardiovascular events related to CAV compared to patients treated with azathioprine (7.9% vs. 13.6%) (Eisen *et al.*, 2006; Keogh *et al.*, 2007).

The available data suggest the efficacy of PSIs in reducing the incidence of CAV; however, up to 30-40% of patients in the clinical trials had to discontinue the PSI during the first year because of poor tolerability. Complications and side effects include bacterial and viral infections (17-30%), oral ulcerations, pericardial effusions (up to 25%) and pleural effusions (15-40%), hematologic abnormalities including anemia and thrombocytopenia, impaired wound healing, acne, and pedal edema. Adverse events may be related to the dosing regimen (high vs. low dose) and timing (immediately post transplant vs. delayed introduction). A recent study with lower serum concentrations of everolimus (3-8ng/mL) report a lower drop-out rate of 15% (Lehmukuhl *et al.*, 2009). At this time, it remains unclear whether patients should be transitioned to a PSI-based immunosuppressant regimen once sternal healing has occurred.

In relation to the pharmacologic treatment of established CAV, aggressive control of traditional cardiac risk factors is important; however, the PSIs represent the most important advance. Studies in which patients with established CAV were switched to a PSI from MMF or azathioprine demonstrated a significant reduction in CAV-related adverse events (5% vs. 25%) including death, percutaneous coronary intervention (PCI), myocardial infarction, or angiographic progression of the disease 2 years following the transition and a reduction in plaque size compared to progression (Mancini *et al.*, 2003; Segovia *et al.*, 2004). Larger studies are needed to corroborate these initial findings; however, it is generally accepted practice that patients with established CAV are transitioned to PSI.

The treatment of established CAV represents a clinical challenge. Non-pharmacologic treatment includes PCI, coronary artery bypass grafting (CABG), and retransplantation. Percutaneous and surgical revascularization is limited by the diffuse coronary involvement, the infrequency of focal lesions with suitable distal targets, and the high mortality rates with surgical intervention (up to 30-40%) (Musci *et al.*, 1998; Patel *et al.*, 1997). PCI is associated with excellent short-term results, however is associated with high restenosis rates. With the advent of drug eluting stents, preliminary studies suggest much lower restenosis rates. (Lee *et al.*, 2008). PCI remains a palliative therapy, as CAV is a diffuse and progressive disease process. It may be appropriate to perform PCI in patients with discrete focal lesions with abnormal graft function or evidence of stress-induced functional significance by stress imaging. Retransplantation is the only definitive therapy for CAV; however, survival is lower than after primary heart transplant and the probability of CAV in the retransplanted heart is higher than in de novo transplants (up to 50% at 3 years) (Musci *et al.*, 1998; Srivastava *et al.*, 2000). Re-transplantation is reserved for highly selected patients with CAV.

9. Summary

The development of CAV has been described as the Achilles heel of cardiac transplantation. The increased mortality observed in the years after the diagnosis of CAV reflects that fact that, at present, the management of these patients represents a clinical challenge. Diagnosis is heavily reliant on invasive testing and early diagnosis and preventive strategies are crucial, but remain ineffective in many cases. Statins, antihypertensive drugs, and anti-CMV agents have all demonstrated a modest beneficial reduction in CAV; however, the proliferation signal inhibitors represent the best prevention and treatment options available at this time. Current research focuses on identification of novel agents that are effective in preventing the development and progression of CAV, and non-invasive techniques for CAV diagnosis.

10. References

Al-Khaldi A, Oyer PE, Robbins RC. (2006). Outcome analysis of donor gender in heart transplantation. *Journal of Heart and Lung Transplantation,* Vol. 25, No. 4, (February 2006), pp. 461-468, ISSN 1053-2498.

Arora S, Gunther A, Wennerblom B, Uelan T, Andreassen AK, Gude E, Endresen K, Geiran O, Wilhelmsen N, Andersen R, Aukrust P, Gullestad L. (2010). Systemic Markers of inflammation are associated with cardiac allograft vasculopathy and an increased intimal inflammatory component. *American Journal of Transplantation,* Vol. 10, No. 6, (June 2010), pp. 1428-1436, ISSN 1600-6135.

Bae JH, Rihal CS, Edwards BS, Kushwaha SS, Mathew V, Prasad A, Holmes DR Jr, Lerman A. (2006). Association of angiotensin-converting enzyme inhibitors and serum lipids with plaque regression in cardiac allograft vasculopathy. *Transplantation,* Vol 82, No. 8, (October 2006), pp. 1108-1111, ISSN 0041-1337.

Bieber CP, Stinson EB, Shumway NE, Payne R, Kosek J. (1970). Cardiac transplantation in man. VII. Cardiac allograft vasculopathy. *Circulation,* Vol. 41, No. 5, (January 1970), pp. 753-72, ISSN 0009-7322.

Briscoe DM , Yeung AC, Schoen FJ, Allred EN, Stavrakis G, Ganz P, Cotran RS, Pober JS, Schoen EL. (1995). Predictive value of inducible endothelial cell adhesion molecule expression for acute rejection of human cardiac allografts. *Transplantation,* Vol. 59, No. 2, (January 1995), pp. 204-211, ISSN 0041-1337.

Cohen O, De La Zerda DJ, Beygui R, Hekmat D, Laks H. (2007). Donor brain death mechanisms and outcomes after heart transplantation. *Transplantation Proceedings,* Vol. 39, No. 10, (December 2007), pp:2964-2969, ISSN 0041-1345.

Costanzo MR, Naftel DC, Pritzker MR, Hellman JK, Boehmer JP, Brozena SC, Dec WG, Ventura HO, Kirklin JK, Bourge RC, Miller LW. (1998). Heart transplant coronary artery disease detected by coronary angiography: a multi-institutional study of preoperative donor and recipient risk factors. Cardiac Transplant Research Database. *The Journal of Heart and Lung Transplantation,* Vol. 17, No. 8, (August 1998), pp744-753, ISSN 1053-2498.

De Marco T, Dae M, Yuen-Green M, Kumar S, Sudhir K, Keith F, Amidon T, Rifkin C, Klinski C, Lau D, Botvinick E, Chatterjee K. (1995). Iodine-123 metaiodobenzylguanidine scintigraphic assessment of the transplanted human heart: evidence for late reinnervation. *Journal of the American College of Cardiology,* Vol. 25, No. 4, (March 1995), pp. 927-931, ISSN 0735-1097.

Derumeaux G, Redonnet M, Mouton-Schleifer D, Bessou JP, Cribier A, Saoudi N, Koning R, Soyer R, Letac B; VACOMED Research Group. (1995). Dobutamine stress echocardiography in orthotopic heart transplant recipients. *Journal of the American College of Cardiology,* Vol. 25, No. 7, (June 1995), pp. 1665-1672, ISSN 0735-1097.

Eisen HJ, Tuzcu EM, Dorent R, Kobashigawa J, Mancini D, Valantine-von Kaeppler HA, Starling RC, Sorensen K, Hummel M, Lind JM, Abeywickrama KH, Bernhardt P. (2003). Everolimus for the prevention of allograft rejection and vasculopathy in cardiac transplant recipients. *New England Journal of Medicine,* Vol. 349, No. 9, (August 2003), pp. 847-858, ISSN 0028-4793.

Eisen H, Yang X. (2006). The impact of proliferation signal inhibitors on the healthcare burden of major adverse cardiac events following heart transplantation. *Transplantation,* Vol. 82, No. 8 SUPPL, (October 2006), pp. S13-18, ISSN 0041-1337.

Ferri C, Properzi G, Tomassoni G, Santucci A, Desideri G, Giuliani AE, Cook DJ, McCarthy P, Young JB, Yamani MH. (2002). Patterns of myocardial endothelin-1 expression and outcome after cardiac transplantation. *Circulation,* Vol. 105, No. 15, (April 2002), pp. 1768-1771, ISSN 0009-7322.

Gasink LB, Blumberg EA, Localio AR, Desai SS, Israni AK, Lautenbach E. (2006). Hepatitis C virus seropositivity in organ donors and survival in heart transplant recipients. *JAMA,* Vol. 296, No. 15, (October 2006), pp. 1843-1850, ISSN 0098-7484

Haji SA, Avery RK, Yamani MH, Tuzcu EM, Crowe TD, Cook DJ, Mawhorter SD, Hobbs R, Young JB, Smedira N, Starling RC. (2006). Donor or recipient hepatitis B seropositivity is associated with allograft vasculopathy. *Journal of Heart and Lung Transplantation,* Vol. 25, No. 3, (March 2006), pp. 294-297, ISSN 1053-2498.

Haji SA, Starling RC, Avery RK, Mawhorter S, Tuzcu EM, Schoenhagen P, Cook DJ, Ratliff NB, McCarthy PM, Young JB, Yamani MH. (2004). Donor hepatitis-C seropositivity is an independent risk factor for the development of accelerated coronary vasculopathy and predicts outcome after cardiac transplantation. *The Journal of Heart and Lung Transplantation,* Vol. 23, No. 3, (March 2004), pp. 277-283, ISSN 1053-2498.

Hollenberg M, Klein LW, Parrillo JE, Scherer M, Burns D, Tamburro P, Oberoi M, Johson MR, Costanzo MR. (2001). Coronary endothelial dysfunction after heart transplantation predicts allograft vasculopathy and cardiac death. *Circulation,* Vol. 104, No. 25, (2001), pp. 3091- 3096, ISSN 0009-7322.

Hosenpud JD, Streblow DN, Kreklywich C, Yin Q, De La Melena VT, Corless CL, Smith PA, Brakebill C, Cook JW, Vink C, Bruggeman CA, Nelson JA, Orloff SL. (2003). Cytomegalovirus-mediated upregulation of chemokine expression correlates with the acceleration of chronic rejection in rat heart transplant. *Journal of Virology,* Vol. 77, No. 3, (February 2003), pp. 2182-2194, ISSN 0022-538X.

Itagaki BK, Kobashigawa JA, Wu GW, Patel JK, Kawano MA, Kittleson MM, Fishbein MC. (2007). Widespread fibrosis of myocardial and adjacent tissues causing restrictive cardiac physiology in patients needing re-do heart transplant. *Proceedings of the International Society of Heart and Lung Transplantation*, San Francisco, April 2007.

Jimenez J, Kapadia SR, Yamani MH, Platt L, Hobbs RE, Rincon G, Botts-Silverman C, Starling R, Young JB, Nissen SE, Tuzcu M. (2001). Cellular rejection and rate of progression of transplant vasculopathy: A 3-year serial intravascular ultrasound study. *Journal of Heart and Lung Transplantation*, Vol. 20, No. 4, (April 2001), pp. 393-398, ISSN 1053-2498.

Kapadia SR, Ziada KM, L'Allier PL, Crowe TD, Rincon G, Hobbs RE, Bott-Silverman C, Young JB, Nissen SE, Tuzcu EM. (2000). Intravascular ultrasound imaging after cardiac transplantation: advantage of multivessel imaging. *The Journal of Heart and Lung Transplantation*, Vol. 19, No. 2, (February 2000), pp. 167-172, ISSN 1053-2498.

Keogh A, Richardson M, Ruygrok P, Spratt P, Galbraith A, O'Driscoll G, Macdonald P, Esmore D, Muller D, Faddy S. (2004). Sirolimus in de novo heart transplant recipients reduces acute rejection and prevents coronary artery disease at 2 years: a randomized clinical trial. *Circulation*, Vol. 110, No. 17, (October 2004), pp. 2694-2700, ISSN 0009-7322.

Keogh A, Richardson M, Ruygrok P, Macdonald P, Schneider L, O'Driscoll G, Galbraith A. (2007). Sirolimus vs. azathioprine from the time of heart transplantation: 65 month follow-up for vascular (MACE) and malignant events. *Proceedings of the International Society of Heart and Lung Transplantation*, San Francisco, April 2007.

Keogl AM, Valantine HA, Hunt SA, Schroeder J, McIntosh N, Oyer P, Stinson E. (1992). Impact of proximal or midvessel discrete coronary artery stenosis on survival after heart transplanation. *The Journal of Heart and Lung Transplantation*, Vol. 11, (1992), pp. 892-901.

Kobashigawa JA, Tobis JM, Starling RC, Tuzcu EM, Smith AL, Valantine HA, Yeung AC, Mehra MR, Anzai H, Oeser BT, Abeywickrama KH, Murphy J, Cretin N. (2005). Multicenter intravascular ultrasound validation study among heart transplant recipients: outcomes after five years. *Journal of the American College of Cardiology*, Vol. 45, No. 9, (May 2005), pp. 1532-1537, ISSN 0735-1097.

Koskinen PK. (1993). The association of the induction of vascular cell adhesion molecule-1 with cytomegalovirus antigenemia in human heart allografts. *Transplantation*, Vol. 56, No. 5, (November 1993), pp. 1103-1108, ISSN 0041-1337.

Labarrere CA, Nelson DR, Cox CJ, Pitts D, Kirlin P, Halbrook H. (2000). Cardiac-specific troponin I levels and risk of coronary artery disease and graft failure following heart transplantation. *Journal of the American Medical Association*, Vol. 284, No. 4, (July 2000), pp. 457-464, ISSN 0098-7484.

Lee MS, Kobashigawa J, Tobis J. (2008). Comparison of percutaneous coronary intervention with bare metal and drug eluting stents for cardiac allograft vasculopathy. *Journal of the American College of Cardiology: Cardiovascular Interventions*, Vol. 1, No. 6, (December 2008), pp. 710-715, ISSN 1936-8798.2282

Lehmukuhl H, Arizon J, Vigano M, Almenar L, Gerosa G, Maccherini M, Varnous S, Musumeci F, Hexham J, Mange K, Livi U. (2009). Everolimus with reduced cyclosporine versus MMF with standard cyclosporine in de novo heart transplant recipients. *Transplantation*, Vol. 88, No. 1, (July 2009), pp. 115-122, ISSN 0041-1337.

Li H, Tanaka K, Anzai H, Oeser B, Lai D, Kobashigawa JA, Tobis JM. (2006). Influence of pre-existing donor atherosclerosis on the development of cardiac allograft vasculopathy and outcomes in heart transplant recipients. *Journal of the American College of Cardiology,* Vol. 47, No. 12, (June 2006), pp. 2470-2476, ISSN 0735-1097.

Libby P, Tanaka H. (1994). The pathogenesis of coronary arteriosclerosis ("chronic rejection") in transplanted hearts. *Clinical Transplantation,* Vol. 3, No. 2 (June 1994), pp. 313-318, ISSN 0902-0063.

Luyt CE, Drobinski G, Dorent R, Ghossoub J, Collet J, Choussat R, Dalby M Thomas D, Gandjbakhch I. (2003). Prognosis of moderate coronary artery lesions in heart transplant patients. *The Journal of Heart and Lung Transplantation,* Vol. 22, No. 2, (February 2003), pp. 130-136, ISSN 1053-2498.

Mancini D, Pinney S, Burkhoff D, LaManca J, Itescu S, Burke E, Edwards N, Oz M, Marks A. (2003). Use of rapamycin slows progression of cardiac transplantation vasculopathy. *Circulation,* Vol. 108, No. 1, (July 2003), pp. 48-53, ISSN 0009-7322.

Martinez-Dolz L, Almenar L, Martinez-Ortiz L, Arnau MA, Chamorro C, Moro J, Osa A, Rueda J, Garcia C, Palencia M. (2005). Predictive factors for development of diabetes mellitus post-heart transplant. *Transplantation Proceedings,* Vol. 37, No. 9, (November 2005), pp. 4064-4066, ISSN 0041-1345.

Mehra MR, Crespo-Leiro MG, Dipchand A, Ensminger SM, Hiemann NE, Kobashigawa JA, Madsen J, Parameshwar J, Starling RC, Uber PA. (2010). International Society for Heart and Lung Transplantation working formulation of a standardized nomenclature for cardiac allograft vasculopathy - 2010. *The Journal of Heart and Lung Transplantation,* Vol. 29, No. 7, (July 2010), pp. 717-727, ISSN 1053-2498.

Mehra MR & Raval NY. (2004c). Metaanalysis of statins and survival in de novo cardiac transplantation. *Transplantation Proceedings,* Vol. 36, No. 5, (June 2004), pp. 1539-1541, ISSN 0041-1345.

Mehra MR, Uber PA, Potluri S, Ventura HO, Scott RL, Park MH. (2004b). Usefulness of an elevated B-type natriuretic peptide to predict allograft failure, cardiac allograft vasculopathy, and survival after heart transplantation. *American Journal of Cardiology,* Vol. 94, No. 4, (August 2004), pp. 454-458, ISSN 0002-9149.

Mehra MR, Uber PA, Ventura HO, Scott RL, Park MH. (2004a). The impact of mode of donor brain death on cardiac allograft vasculopathy. *Journal of the American College of Cardiology,* Vol. 43, No. 5, (March 2004), pp. 806-810, ISSN 0735-1097.

Mehra MR, Ventura HO, Stapleton DD, Smart FW, Collins TC, Ramee SR. (1995). Presence of severe intimal thickening by intravascular ultrasonography predicts cardiac events in cardiac allograft vasculopathy. *The Journal of Heart and Lung Transplantation,* Vol. 14, No. 4, (July-August 1995), pp. 632-639, ISSN 1053-2498.

Michaels PJ, Espejo ML, Kobashigawa J, Alejos JC, Burch C, Takemoto S, Reed EF, Fishbein MC. (2003). Humoral rejection in cardiac transplantation: risk factors, hemodynamic consequences and relationship to transplant coronary artery disease. *Journal of Heart and Lung Transplantation,* Vol. 22, No. 1, (January 2003), pp. 58-69, ISSN 1053-2498.

Muehling OM, Wilke NM, Panse P, Jerosch-Herold M, Wilson BV, Wilson RF, Miller LW. (2003). Reduced myocardial perfusion reserve and transmural perfusion gradient in heart transplant arteriopathy assessed by magnetic resonance imaging. *Journal of the American College of Cardiology,* Vol. 42, No. 6, (September 2003), pp.1054-1060, ISSN 0735-1097.

Musci M, Loebe M, Wellnhofer E, Meyer R, Pasic M, Hummel M, Bocksch W, Grauhan O, Weng Y, Hetzer R. (1998). Coronary angioplasty, bypass surgery, and retransplantation in cardiac transplant patients with graft coronary artery disease. *The Journal of Thoracic and Cardiovascular Surgery*, Vol. 46, No. 5, (October 1998), pp. 268-274, ISSN 0171-6425.

Nagji AS, Hranjec T, Swenson BR, Kern JA, Bergin JD, Jones DR, Kron IL, Lau CL, Ailawadi G. (2010). Donor age is associated with chronic allograft vasculopathy after adult heart transplantation: implications for donor allocation. *Annals of Thoracic Surgery*, Vol. 90, No. 1, (July 2010), pp. 168-175, ISSN 0003-4975.

Neish AS, Loh E, Schoen FJ. (1992). Myocardial changes in cardiac transplant-associated coronary arteriosclerosis: potential for timely diagnosis. *Journal of the American College of Cardiology*, Vol. 19, No. 3, (March 1992), pp.586-592, ISSN 0735-1097.

Nissen S. (2001). Coronary angiography and intravascular ultrasound. *American Journal of Cardiology*, Vol. 87, No. 4A, (February 2001), pp. 15A-20A, ISSN 0002-9149.

Novitzky D, Rose AG, Cooper DK. (1988). Injury of myocardial conduction tissue and coronary artery smooth muscle following brain death in the baboon. *Transplantation*, Vol. 45, No. 5, (May 1988), pp. 964-966, ISSN 0041-1337.

Pardo Mindan FJ, Panizo A, Lozano MD, Herreros J, Mejia S. (1997). Role of endomyocardial biopsy in the diagnosis of chronic rejection in human heart transplantation. *Clinical Transplantation*, Vol. 11, No. 5, (October 1997), pp. 426-431, ISSN 0902-0063.

Patel VS, Radovancevic B, Springer W, Frazier OH, Massin E, Benrey J, Kadipasaoglu K, Cooley DA. (2007). Revascularization procedures in patients with transplant coronary artery disease. *European Journal of Cardiothoracic Surgery*, Vol. 11, No. 5, (May 1997), pp. 895-901, ISSN 1010-7940.

Pflugfelder PW, Boughner DR, Rudas L, Kostuk WJ. (1993). Enhanced detection of cardiac allograft arterial disease with intracoronary ultrasonographic imaging. *American Heart Journal*, Vol. 125, No. 6, (June 1993), pp. 1583-1591, ISSN 0002-8703.

Potena L & Valantine H. (2007). Cardiac allograft vasculopathy and insulin resistance - hope for new therapeutic targets. *Endocrinology and Metabolism Clinics of North America*, Vol. 36, No. 4, (December 2007), pp. 965-981, ISSN 0889-8529.

Raichlin E, Edwards BS, Kremers WK, Clavell AL, Rodeheffer RJ, Frantz RP, Pereira NL, Daly RC, McGregor CG, Lerman A, Kushwaha SS. (2009). Acute cellular rejection and the subsequent development of allograft vasculopathy after cardiac transplantation. *Journal of Heart and Lung Transplantation*, Vol. 28, No. 4, (April 2009), pp. 320-327, ISSN 1053-2498.

Raichlin ER, McConnell JP, Lerman A, Kremers WK, Edwards BS, Kushwaha SS, Clavell AL, Rodeheffer RJ, Frantz RP. (2007). Systemic inflammation and metabolic syndrome in cardiac allograft vasculopathy. *Journal of Heart and Lung Transplantation*, Vol. 26, No. 8. (August 2007), pp. 826-833, ISSN 1053-2498.

Rickenbacher PR, Pinto FJ, Lewis NP, Hunt SA, Alderman EL, Schroeder JS, Stinson EB, Brown BW, Valantine HA. (1995). Prognostic importance of intimal thickness as measured by intracoronary ultrasound after cardiac transplantation. *Circulation*, Vol. 92, No. 12, (December 1995), pp. 3445-3452, ISSN 0009-7322.

Sanchez Lazaro IJ, Bonet LA, Lopez JM, Lacuesta ES, Martinez-Dolz L, Ramon-Llin J,A Lalaguna LA, Perez OC, Martinez VO, Fuentes FB, Sanz AS. (2008). Influence of traditional cardiovascular risk factors in the recipient on the development of cardiac allograft vasculopathy after heart transplantation. *Transplantation Proceedings*, Vol. 40, No. 9, (November 2008), pp. 3056 - 3057, ISSN 0041-1345.

Schepis T, Achenbach S, Weyand M, Raum P, Marwan M, Pflederer T, Daniel WB, Tandler R, Kondruweit M, Ropers D. (2009). Comparison of dual source computed tomography versus intravascular ultrasound for evaluation of coronary arteries at least one year after cardiac transplantation. *American Journal of Cardiology*, Vol. 104, No. 10, (November 2009), pp. 1351-1356, ISSN 0002-9149.

Schoreder JS, Gao SZ, Alderman EL, Hunt SA, Johnstone I, Boothroyd DB, Wiederhold V, Stinson EB. (1993). A preliminary study of diltiazem in the prevention of coronary artery disease in heart-transplant recipients. *New England of Journal of Medicine*, Vol. 328, No. 3, (January 1993), pp. 164-170, ISSN 0028-4793.

Segel LD, Von Haag DW, Zhang J, Follette DM. (2002). Selective overexpression of inflammatory molecules in hearts from brain-dead rats. *Journal of Heart and Lung Transplantation*, Vol. 21, No. 7, July 2002), pp. 804-811, ISSN 1053-2498.

Segovia J, Aloinso-Pulpon L, Ortiz P, Jimenez-Mazuecos J, Alfonso F, Escaned J, Hernandez-Antolin R, Macaya C. (2004). Rapastat: evaluation of the role of oral sirolimus in the treatment of established graft vessel disease. A prospective, randomized intravascular ultrasound study. *Proceedings from the International Society of Heart and Lung* Transplantation, San Francisco, April 2004.

Spes CH, Klauss V, Mudra H, Schnaack SD, Tammen AR, Rieber J, Siebert U, Henneke KH, Uberfuhr P, Reichart B, Theisen K, Angermann CE. (1999). Diagnostic and prognostic value of serial dobutamine stress echocardiography for noninvasive assessment of cardiac allograft vasculopathy: a comparison with coronary angiography and intravascular ultrasound. *Circulation*, Vol. 100, No. 5, (August 1999), pp. 509-515, ISSN 0009-7322.

Srivastava R, Keck BM, Bennett LE, Hosenpud JD. (2000). The results of cardiac retransplantation: an analysis of the Joint International Society for Heart and Lung Transplantation/United Network for Organ Sharing Thoracic Registry. *Transplantation*, Vol. 70, No. 4, pp. 606-612, ISSN 0041-1337.

Stork S, Behr T, Birk M, Uberfuhr P, Klauss V, Spes C, Angermann C. (2006). Assessment of cardiac allograft vasculopathy late after heart transplantation: when is coronary angiography necessary? *The Journal of Heart and Lung Transplantation*, Vol. 25, No. 9, (September 2006), pp. 1103-1108, ISSN 1053-2498.

Takada M, Nadeau KC, Hancock WW, Mackenzie HS, Shaw GD, Waaga AM, Chandraker A, Sayegh MH, Tilney NL. (1998). Effects of explosive brain death on cytokine activation of peripheral organs in the rat. *Transplantation*, Vol. 65, No. 12, (June 1998), pp. 1533-1542, ISSN 0041-1337.

Taylor DO, Edwards LB, Boucek MM, Trulock EP, Waltz, DA, Keck BM, Hertz MI. (2006). Registry of the International Society for Heart and Lung Transplantation: twenty-third official adult heart transplantation report - 2006. *The Journal of Heart and Lung Transplantation*, Vol. 25, No. 8, (August 2006), pp. 869-879, ISSN 1053-2498.

Taylor DO , Edwards LB, Boucek MM, Trulock EP, Aurora P, Christie J, Dobbels F, Rahmel AO, Keck BM, Hertz MI. (2007). Registry of the International Society for Heart and Lung Transplantation: twenty-fourth official heart transplant report -2007. *Journal of Heart and Lung Transplantation*, Vol. 26, No. 8, (August 2007), pp. 769-781, ISSN 1053-2498.

Tona F, Caforio A, Montisci R, Gambino A, Angelini A, Ruscazio M, toscano G, Feltrin F, Ramondo A, Gerosa G, Iliceto S. (2006). Coronary Flow Velocity Pattern and Coronary Flow Reserve by Contrast-Enhanced Transthoracic echocardiography predict long-term outcome in heart transplantation. *Circulation*, Vol. 114, No. I Suppl, (July 2006), pp. I49-I55, ISSN 0009-7322.

Tsutsui H, Ziada KM, Schoenhagen P, Iyisoy A, Magyar WA, Crowe TD, Klingensmith JD, Vince DG, Rincon G, Hobbs RE, Yamagishi M, Nissen SE, Tuzcu EM. (2001). Lumen loss in transplant coronary artery disease is a biphasic process involving early intimal thickening and late constrictive remodeling: results from a 5-year serial intravascular ultrasound study. *Circulation*, Vol. 104, No. 6, pp. 653-657, ISSN 0009-7322.

Tuzcu EM, Kapadia SR, Sachar R, Ziada KM, Crowe TD, Feng J, Magyar WA, Hobbs RE, Starling RC, Young JB, McCarthy P, Nissen SE. (2005). Intravascular ultrasound evidence of angiographically silent progression in coronary atherosclerosis predicts long-term morbidity and mortality after cardiac transplantation. *Journal of the American College of Cardiology*, Vol. 45, No. 9, (May 2005), pp. 1538-1542, ISSN 0735-1097.

Valantine HA, Gao SZ, Menon SG, Renlund DG, Hunt SA, Oyer P, Stinson EB, Brown BW, Merigan TC, Schroeder JS. (1999). Impact of prophylactic immediate posttransplant ganciclovir on development of transplant atherosclerosis: A post hoc analysis of a randomized, placebo-controlled study. *Circulation*, Vol. 100, No. 1, (July 1999), pp. 61-66, ISSN 0009-7322.

Valantine H, Rickenbacker P, Kemna M, Hunt S, Chen Y, Reaven G, Stinson E. (2001). Metabolic abnormalities characteristic of dysmetabolic syndrome predict the development of transplant coronary artery disease: a prospective study. *Circulation*, Vol. 103, No. 17, (May 2001), pp. 2144-2152, ISSN 0009-7322.

Van Dorp WT, Jonges E, Bruggeman CA, Daha MR, Van Es LA, Van Der Woude FJ. (1989). Direct induction of MHC class I, but not class II, expression on endothelial cells by cytomegalovirus infection. *Transplantation*, Vol. 48, No. 3, (September 1989), pp. 469-472, ISSN 0041-1337.

We GW, Kobashigawa JA, Fishbein MC, Patel JK, Kittleson MM, Reed EF, Kiyosaki KK, Ardehali A. (2009). Asymptomatic antibody-mediated rejection after heart transplantation predicts poor outcomes. *Journal of Heart and Lung Transplantation*, Vol. 28, No. 5, (May 2009), pp. 417-422, ISSN 1053-2498.

Weill D. (2001). Role of cytomegalovirus in cardiac allograft vasculopathy. *Transplant Infectious Disease*, Vol. 3, Supplement 2, (2001), pp. 44-48, ISSN 1398-2273.

Weis, M, Kledal TN, Lin KY, Panchal SN, Gao SZ, Valantine HA, Mocarski ES, Cooke JP. (2004). Cytomegalovirus infection impairs the nitric oxide synthase pathway: role of asymmetric dimethylarginine in transplant arteriosclerosis. *Circulation*, Vol. 109, No. 4, (February 2004), pp. 500-505, ISSN 0009-7322.

Wenke K, Meiser B, Thiery J, Nagel D, von Scheidt W, Krobot K, Steinbeck G, Seidel D, Reichart B. (2003). Simvastatin initiated early after heart transplantation: 8-year prospective experience. *Circulation*, Vol. 107, No. 1, (January 2003), pp. 93-97, ISSN 0009-7322.

Yamasaki M, Sakurai R, Hirohata A, Honda Y, Bonneau HN, Luikart H, Yock PG, Fitzgerald PJ, Yeung AC, Valantine HA, Fearon WF. (2011). Impact of donor-transmitted atherosclerosis on early cardiac allograft vasculopathy: new findings by three-dimensional intravascular ultrasound analysis. *Transplantation,* Vol. 91, No. 12, (June 2011), pp. 1406-1411, ISSN 0041-1337.

6

Role of Matricellular Proteins in Cardiac Allograft Fibrosis

Nadine Frerker*, Monika Kasprzycka*, Bjørg Mikalsen,
Pål Dag Line, Helge Scott and Guttorm Haraldsen
*Dept. and Inst. Of Pathology, Dept of Surgery,
Oslo University Hospital and University of Oslo, Oslo,
Norway*

1. Introduction

While acute rejection of solid organ allografts has become a rare clinical condition, long-term graft survival is threatened by the development of fibrosis. Such fibrosis is seen in two forms in the heart, one being an accelerated process of atherosclerosis termed transplant vasculopathy, the second a parenchymal response to the ensuing ischemia, low-grade cellular or humoral allorejection, as well as other factors.

The transplant vasculopathy (TV) of cardiac allografts (also known as graft vascular disease, chronic allograft vasculopathy or graft vascular sclerosis) is defined as a diffuse proliferative process that causes obstruction of the coronary vasculature, impairment of vascular flow and secondary myocardial ischemic injury (Mitchell, 2009). Whereas atherosclerosis of non-transplanted hearts mainly affects the proximal part of the coronary arteries, TV affects the arteries down to the level of small intramyocardial branches. Moreover, similar but less extensive changes have been observed in coronary veins (Mitchell, 2009), whereas changes in capillary basement membrane structure, as seen in chronic kidney rejection biopsies, have not been identified as a feature of chronic rejections in hearts.

The TV lesion consists of concentric intimal thickening that contains modified smooth muscle cells that have most likely migrated from the media, macrophages that contain intracellular lipids, collagen and glycosoaminoglycans (Winters & Schoen, 2001). Cholesterol clefts in a band-like distribution and lesions resembling typical atheromatous plaques may arise in the advanced form of the disease. The endothelium and internal elastic lamina are nearly always intact. The vascular media may have normal thickness or may be thinned. Cellular infiltrates, including T-lymphocytes, both CD4+ and CD8+, and macrophages are frequently present as a superficial band in the subendothelium and deeper within the intima and media.

On the other hand, interstitial fibrosis is also a feature of transplanted hearts, partly a consequence of the ischemia associated with TV, but also total ischemic time, rejection episodes and donor cause of death. Despite these different origins of graft fibrosis, the fibrosis lesion (including intimafibrosis in TV) appears to have the occurrence of myofibroblasts or myofibroblast-like cells in common. Myofibroblasts are contractile cells thought to partly derive from fibroblasts and to share characteristics with smooth muscle cells, including expression of α-smooth muscle actin (SMA). They play an important role in physiologic wound healing by synthesizing collagens and exerting strong contraction forces to minimize wound areas (comprehensive reviews of myofibroblast origins, differentiation and functions can be found in (Hinz, 2010; Wipff & Hinz, 2009). Their recruitment is thought to be mediated by cellular damage, the release of inflammatory mediators including TLR agonists (Wynn, 2008).

2. Matricellular proteins – between cell and matrix

The ECM consists of a complex network of structural proteins (collagens, elastin), multidomain adhesive glycoproteins (fibronectin, vitronectin, and laminin), glycosaminoglycans (GAGs) such as hyaluronan and proteoglycans (versican, syndecans, glypicans, perlecan), as well as the matricellular proteins that we shall focus on in this chapter.

Although the main role of ECM is to act as a structural scaffold for tissue and a compression buffer when tissues are subjected to stress, its ability to also provide the contextual information responsible for controlling cellular behaviour has been increasingly recognized in recent years. The biophysical properties of the matrix can regulate cellular mechanosensory pathways - through global substrate rigidity or extracellular tension. Specific domains and motifs embedded in the ECM proteins act as ligands for cellular receptors, such as integrins and discoidin domain tyrosine kinase receptors. In addition, the ECM also sequesters and hence acts as a reservoir for a wide range of growth factors and cytokines (for reviews see Cox & Erler, 2011; Hynes, 2009; Rhodes & Simons, 2007; Schultz & Wysocki, 2009).

Matricellular protein is a term originally proposed by Bornstein (Bornstein, 1995) to describe secreted extracellular matrix proteins that function more as regulators of cell-matrix interactions than as structural proteins. The group of matricellular proteins includes amongst others thrombospondins, tenascins, osteopontin, periostin, osteonectin or CCN proteins. A common property of matricellular proteins is their high expression level during embryogenesis, which is strongly reduced after birth and becomes low to absent in adult life (although there are organ specific differences). Their expression re-appears at high levels in response to tissue injury (Bornstein & Sage, 2002).

2.1 Osteopontin

Osteopontin (also known as 44kDa bone phosphoprotein, sialoprotein I, secreted phosphoprotein I, uropontin, and early T lymphocyte activation-1) is a multifunctional protein thought to play a significant role in a variety of biological processes, including bone resorption, immune cell activation, atherosclerosis and ECM remodeling (Scatena et al., 2007). It belongs to the small integrin binding ligand N-linked glycoprotein (SIBLING) family-related proteins. It is composed of 314 amino acid residues and is subject to profound posttranslational modifications such as phosphorylation and glycosylation (Waller et al., 2010). Osteopontin has several molecular domains of established or putative function (see Firgure), among them several integrin binding domains: an arginine-glycine-aspartic acid (RGD) cell binding sequence interacts with integrins αvβ3, αvβ1, αvβ5 and α8β1, a serine-

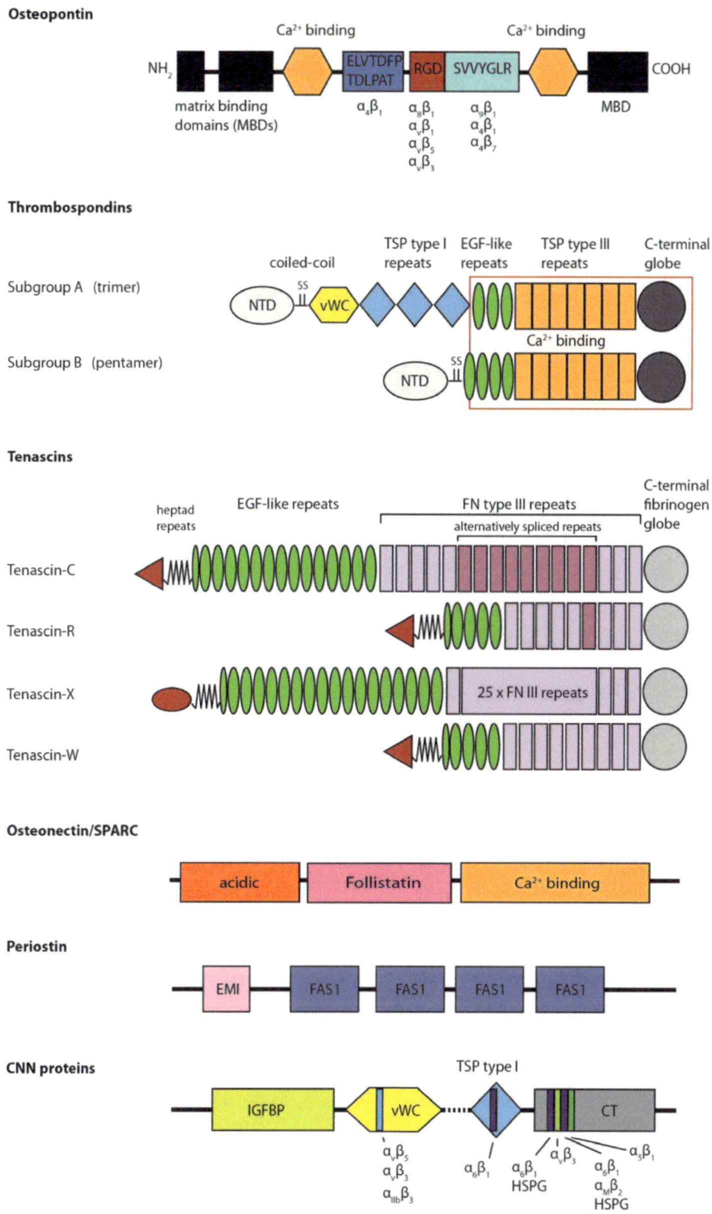

Fig. 1. Structural models of matricellular proteins.
Osteopontin: MBD = matrix binding domain, the integrin binding specificity is indicated below corresponding domains; *Thrombospondins*: NTD = N-terminal domain, vWC = von Willebrand factor type C domain, TSP = thrombospondin, red box indicates conserved domains, *Tenascins*: in red = N-terminal oligomerisation domain, FN = fibronectin; *Osteonectin* with the three characteristic domains of SPARC-like proteins; *Periostin*: FAS1 domain = fasciclin-like domain 1; *CCN proteins*:; IGFBP = insulin-like growth factor binding protein homology domain, CT = C-terminal domain, HSPG = heparan sulfate proteoglycan, integrin and HSPG binding sites are indicated in colored bars, dashed line indicates the hinge region (adapted from publications Adams & Lawler, 2004; Brekken & Sage, 2000; C. C. Chen & Lau, 2009; Chiquet-Ehrismann & Chiquet, 2003; Conway & Molkentin, 2008; Lund et al., 2009; Scatena et al., 2007).

valine-valine-tyrosine- glutamate-leucine-arginine (SVVYGLR)-containing domain that interacts with integrins α9β1, α4β1 and α4β7 and a ELVTDFPTDLPAT domain is also reported to bind to α4β1 (Waller et al., 2010). Several cell types have the capacity to synthesize osteopontin, including bone cells, macrophages, endothelial cells, smooth muscle cells and fibroblasts (Schellings et al., 2004). In healthy adult organs osteopontin expression is low except for the kidney, bone, and in epithelial linings of several tissues (Schellings et al., 2004). By contrast, osteopontin expression is upregulated in pathological conditions, such as atherosclerosis (Giachelli et al., 1993) and ischemic injury (Ellison et al., 1998) including myocardial infarction (MI) (Tamura et al., 2003).

2.2 Thrombospondins

The known vertebrate thrombospondins fall into two subgroups, termed A (thrombospondin-1 and -2) and B (thrombospondin-3, -5, and -5/COMP) according to their oligomerization status. Hence, members of subgroup A form homotrimers and members of subgroup B homopentamers. Each thrombospondin contains multiple domains and a coiled-coil oligomerisation region (Figure). The hallmark of all thrombospondins is the presence in the carboxy-terminal half of each polypeptide of a variable number of EGF-like domains that are contiguous with seven so-called thrombospondin type 3 repeats and a C-terminal region of globular character (Adams & Lawler, 2004).

The most well described members of the family are thrombospondin-1 and -2. Important functions of thrombospondin-1 are activation of the TGF-β (transforming growth factor-β, see below), inhibition of angiogenesis and de-adhesion of cells. The anti-angiogenic effect of thrombospondin-1 is caused mostly by induction of apoptosis and inhibition of endothelial cell migration (Nor et al., 2000). Thrombospondin-1 also induces de-adhesion , defined as transition to an earlier stage of adhesion process (Greenwood & Murphy-Ullrich, 1998), in a variety of cells, by stimulating loss of focal adhesions and actin stress fibers (Greenwood & Murphy-Ullrich, 1998; Murphy-Ullrich & Hook, 1989). Likewise, thrombospondin-2 has been shown also to inhibit angiogenesis and cause de-adhesion by inhibiting focal adhesion in endothelial cells (Murphy-Ullrich et al., 1993, for review see Schellings et al., 2004).

2.3 Tenascins

The tenascin family includes: tenascin-C, -R, -X, -Y and -W. They are all built from a common set of structural motifs: heptad repeats, EGF-like repeats, fibronectin type III repeats and a fibrinogen globe domain (FBG, see Figure). At the N-terminus each tenascin has an oligomerisation domain that in the case of tenascin-C and -W leads to the formation of hexamers while tenascin-R has been isolated as a trimeric molecule (Racanelli et al., 1992).

Tenascin-C expression is very low after birth and in the normal adult heart its expression is limited to the chorda tendinae of papillary muscles (Sato & Shimada, 2001). However, the protein reappears under pathological conditions, such as infection, vascular hypertension, myocardial infarction and experimental autoimmune myocarditis (Imanaka-Yoshida et al., 2001; Imanaka-Yoshida et al., 2002). Tenascin-C has adhesive and de-adhesive properties, depending on ECM composition and cell surface receptor binding. De-adhesion facilitates cell migration and tissue remodeling during wound healing. In contrast to tenascin-C, tenascin-X expression remains high after birth (Geffrotin et al., 1995) and has been shown to mediate cell adhesion but not spreading (Elefteriou et al., 1999) Moreover, tenascin-X modulates collagen fibrillogenesis and is therefore described in more detail below.

2.4 Osteonectin/SPARC

Osteonectin (also known as SPARC (Secreted Protein Acidic and Rich in Cysteine) or BM-40) is a 32-kDa glycoprotein characterized by three modular domains (Figure): (1) an N-terminal acidic and low-affinity calcium-binding domain; (2) a disulfide-bonded, copper-binding follistatin domain (homologous to the TGFβ-inhibitors activin and inhibin), and (3) the C-terminal extracellular calcium-binding domain (Clark et al., 1997; Schellings et al., 2004).

Tissue expression of osteonectin in healthy adult organs is very low except in epithelia that exhibit high turnover rates (gut, skin, and glandular tissue) (Sage et al., 1989). However, like the preceding matricellular proteins, osteonectin expression re-appears in lesions of injury such as myocardial infarction (Komatsubara et al., 2003). Osteonectin has been reported to bind to thrombospondin-1, vitronectin, entactin, fibrillar collagens and collagen type IV (Schellings et al., 2004). Additionally, it inhibits endothelial cell adhesion and proliferation (Rosenblatt et al., 1997). The de-adhesive effect is mediated through a tyrosine phosphorylation-dependent pathway, whereas its antiproliferative function is dependent, in part, on signal transduction via a G protein-coupled receptor (Motamed & Sage, 1998). Absence of osteonectin in mice during embryogenesis resulted in pups with curly tails and reduced tensile strength of the skin. Smaller collagen fibrils that were more uniform in diameter were seen at the ultrastructural level (Schellings et al., 2004).

2.5 Periostin

Periostin (osteoblast specific factor-2, OSF-2) (reviewed in refs. Conway & Molkentin, 2008; Norris et al., 2009) has a molecular weight of ~90 kDa and consists of), four-coiled fasciclin-like repeats, an aminoterminal cysteine-rich region (EMI domain), and heparin binding domains present in the carboxyl tail (Figure). In the heart, periostin is expressed at the very early stages of embryogenesis; however, it is not detected in the normal adult myocardium, except in the valves (Kruzynska-Frejtag et al., 2001; Norris et al., 2007).

Periostin can directly interact with other ECM proteins such as fibronectin, tenascin-C, collagen I, collagen V, and heparin and serve as a ligand for integrins αvβ3, αvβ5 and α4β6. Recently, it was demonstrated that periostin plays a crucial role in activation of fibroblasts and smooth muscle cells (SMC) through FAK-integrin signaling (Li et al., 2010; Shimazaki et al., 2008). It also promotes collagen fibril formation (Maruhashi et al., 2010; Norris et al., 2007) and incorporation of tenascin-C, organizing a meshwork architecture of the ECM (Kii et al., 2010).

2.6 CCN protein family

CCN (an acronym formed from names of first three members) proteins family (reviewed in Chen & Lau, 2009; Kular et al., 2011) includes 6 members: CYR61 (cysteine-rich 61; CCN1), CTGF (connective tissue growth factor; CCN2), NOV (nephroblastoma over-expressed; CCN3), CCN4 (WISP1), CCN5 (WISP2), and CCN6 (WISP3). All members share a multimodular structure, with an N-terminal secretory signal sequence followed by four conserved domains with homology to insulin-like growth factor binding proteins (IGFBPs), von Willebrand factor type C repeat (VWC), thrombospondin type I repeat (TSP) and a carboxyterminal domain (CT) containing a cystein knot (with the exception of CCN5, see figure). A multimodular structure of the CCN proteins allows them to bind and interact with a broad range of partners including integrins, heparan sulfate proteoglycans (HSPGs), ECM components such as fibronectin and fibulin 1C, receptors like Notch1, TrkA, low-density lipoprotein receptor-related proteins (LRPs), growth factors including BMPs, TGF-β and VEGF, as well as gap junction protein connexin 43. CCN proteins regulate cellular functions such as adhesion, migration, proliferation, differentiation, survival, apoptosis or extracellular matrix remodelling in a cell-type specific manner and they play crucial roles in vascular and skeletal development, angiogenesis, wound healing, fibrosis, vascular disease or cancer.

3. Matricellular proteins in action

3.1 Matricellular proteins in solid organ transplantation

Data on matricellular protein expression and function in the cardiac allografts is limited (Franz et al., 2010; Mikalsen et al., 2010; Zhao et al., 2001) but justifies further investigation. For example, TV has been associated with elevated levels of thrombospondin-1 (Zhao et al., 2001) and of tenascin-C (Franz et al., 2010). Moreover, the tenet of endothelial cell activation being at the epicentre of TV pathogenesis leads to the logic that we need a focussed understanding of how this cell type responds without the confounding noise generated from other cell types. Initial studies in our lab were therefore founded on the purification of endothelial cells from heterotopic cardiac grafts in the rat during rejection (Mikalsen et al., 2010). Grafts were fully mismatched (DA to Lewis), leading to a full rejection and loss of graft function at day 5-6, and were compared to isografts (Lewis to Lewis) to discriminate allogenicity from the surgical procedure. The extent of this analysis is a transcriptome-wide, Affymetrix-based profile of rejection on day 2, 3 and 4 and a corresponding profile of the isograft. Among the most interesting features of these profiles was, first, the observation that tenascin-C and periostin were the most strongly induced transcripts and, second, that the majority of transcriptional changes were similar between the allo- and isografts. These data are publicly available at the NCBI GeneExpression Omnibus (**GSE16695).**

Another observation of relevance is that cyclosporine and tacrolimus have been shown to induce osteopontin mRNA expression in renal tissues *in vitro* and *in vivo* (Khanna, 2005). Cyclosporine has been reported to induce upregulation of osteopontin by tubular epithelial cells resulting in macrophage infiltration and fibrosis in a rat model of chronic cyclosporine nephropathy. Whether these findings have an impact on cardiac allografts is uncertain. It appears that cyclosporine does not promote clinical TV (Gamba, Mammana, Fiocchi, Iamele, & Mamprin, 2000; Rickenbacher et al., 1996), despite a large amount of experimental data suggesting a profibrotic effect, including enhanced production of TGF-β.

In addition, Sawada and coworkers studied the role of tenascin-C during abdominal aorta-to-carotid artery interposition grafting in mice (Fischer, 2007; Sawada et al., 2007). When aortas derived from tenasin-C-deficient mice were grafted to carotid arteries of tenascin-C-deficient recipients, neointimal hyperplasia and VSMC proliferation was significantly reduced compared with WT-to-WT grafting. Furthermore, even if only the graft or the recipient was tenascin-C-deficient, dramatic reductions of neointimal hyperplasia occurred.

3.2 Matricellular proteins in ischemic injury

Given that data on matricellular protein expression and function in cardiac allograft fibrosis is currently very limited, it is interesting to look at the role of these proteins in cardiac healing and remodeling after experimental MI. Interestingly, lack of several matricellular proteins reveals remarkable phenotypes in this context (for review see Matsui et al., 2010), most of them (with the exception of thrombospondin-1) showing signs of reduced repair and resulting ventricular dilation.

Thus, osteopontin-deficient mice show significantly stronger ventricular dilation, reduced collagen synthesis and deposition in both infarcted and non-infarcted regions compared to wild-type (WT) mice (Trueblood et al., 2001). Moreover, expression and activity of MMP-2 and MMP-9 is significantly higher in the non-infarct LV in mice lacking osteopontin 3 days post-MI. The increased MMP-2 activity in the KO group persisted over the next 14 days suggesting that osteopontin modulates MMP expression and activity in the heart post-MI, thereby playing an important role in regulation of collagen deposition and fibrosis. While MMP inhibition improved heart function in both WT and KO mice, this improvement was significantly higher in mice lacking osteopontin (Krishnamurthy et al., 2009). Thus, it appears that increased osteopontin expression protects the heart from ventricular dilation and is required to maintain the structure and function of the heart after ischemic injury.

Moreover, thrombospondin-1-deficient mice exhibit severe inflammation and expansion of the ischemic lesion, as well as enhanced ventricular dilatation (Frangogiannis et al., 2005), whereas thrombospondin-2-deficient mice developed cardiac failure in response to angiotensin II infusion, followed by fatal cardiac rupture in 70% of the cohort. Wild-type controls showed no signs of cardiac failure (Schroen et al., 2004).

Likewise, a targeted inactivation of osteonectin exhibited an increased incidence of cardiac rupture and failure after MI, resulting in a fourfold increase in mortality. Ostonectin-null infarcts had a disorganized granulation tissue and immature collagenous ECM. In contrast, adenoviral overexpression of osteonectin in WT mice improved the collagen maturation and prevented cardiac dilatation and dysfunction (Schellings et al., 2009).

In a similar manner, periostin-deficient mice have an increased incidence of cardiac rupture following experimental MI, associated with decreased recruitment of myofibroblasts and impaired collagen fiber formation in the lesion. However, surviving periostin-deficient mice have less fibrosis and significantly better cardiac performance (Matsui et al., 2010; Oka et al., 2007; Shimazaki et al., 2008).

By contrast, the effect of tenascin-C depletion on cardiac healing and remodeling after experimental MI was that end-diastolic pressure, ventricle dimension and myocardial stiffness were less increased of KO+MI compared to WT+MI mice (Nishioka et al., 2010). Histological examination revealed normal tissue healing, but interstitial fibrosis in the residual myocardium of the peri-infarcted areas was significantly less pronounced in KO+MI mice than in WT+MI mice (Nishioka et al., 2010), perhaps due to the delayed appearance of myofibroblast in tenascin-C-deficient mice (Tamaoki et al., 2005).

3.3 Effect of matricellular proteins in the inflammatory response

Given that atherosclerosis, TV, cellular and humoral rejection as all chronic inflammatory conditions, it deserves focus to also discuss the role of matricellular proteins in this context.

3.3.1 Osteopontin

Osteopontin affects inflammatory responses at many different levels (reviewed in Lund et al., 2009 and Scatena et al., 2007). First, osteopontin plays a crucial key role in macrophage biology by regulating migration, survival, phagocytosis, and pro-inflammatory cytokine production *in vitro* (Lund et al., 2009; Weber et al., 2002). Conversely, osteopontin is induced by several inflammatory cytokines in macrophages, including TNF-α, IL-1β, IFN-γ, and IL-6, and other factors such as angiotensin-II, oxidizedLDL, and phorbol-ester (Lund et al., 2009). In CD4+ and CD8+ lymphocytes, osteopontin is strongly induced in response to T cell receptor ligation (Shinohara et al., 2005). *In vivo*, subcutaneous injection of ostopontin leads to recruitment of macrophages (Giachelli et al., 1998) and in osteopontin-deficient mice, macrophage infiltration is greatly diminished compared to wild-type mice in both acute and chronic inflammation models such as unilateral uretheral obstruction (UUO) model (Ophascharoensuk et al., 1999) or type II collagen antibody-induced arthritis (Yumoto et al., 2002). Osteopontin has also been also reported to regulate T cells migration, adhesion, co-stimulation and proliferation (O'Regan et al., 1999; Patarca et al., 1993) as well as migration of neutrophils (Koh et al., 2007) and dendritic cells (Weiss et al., 2001). Moreover, osteopontin can modulate the immune response by enhancing expression of Th1 cytokines by promoting expression of IL-12 and inhibiting that of IL-10 (Ashkar et al., 2000). In addition, there is evidence that matrix degrading enzymes are affected, as matrix metalloprotease (MMP)-2 and MMP-9 activity was reduced after angiotensin II infusion in osteopontin KO mice (Bruemmer et al., 2003) and macrophages stimulated with osteopontin *in vitro* upregulated activated MMP-9 (Weber et al., 2002).

3.3.2 Tenascin C

Midwood and coworkers reported recently that tenascin-C, acting as an endogenous activator of TLR4-mediated immunity, mediates persistent synovial inflammation and tissue destruction in arthritic joint disease (Midwood et al., 2009). *In vitro*, TLR4 ligation also stimulated synthesis of TNF-α, IL-6 and IL-8 in primary human macrophages and IL-6 in synovial fibroblasts. TLR4-binding has been mapped to the FBG domain of tenascin-C at the carboxy terminus of the molecule. Interestingly, tenascin-C does not seem to be involved in the initiation of inflammation but it is required for the maintenance of joint inflammation, perhaps reflecting that it is absent from healthy tissue and needs induction by inflammatory mediators (Goh et al., 2010). The key role of tenascin-C in prolonging joint inflammation was underscored by the protection of tenasin C-/- mice from sustained and erosive joint inflammation (Midwood et al., 2009). Tenascin C can also stimulate cytokine synthesis in murine synovial fibroblasts via activation of α9 integrins (Kanayama et al., 2009).

Moreover, tenascin-C appears to be involved in regulation of lymphocyte migration as it supports adhesion and rolling of primary human peripheral blood and tonsillar lymphocytes (Clark et al., 1997). In addition, tenascin-C KO mice exhibit reduced lymphocyte infiltration and lower levels of IFN, TNF and IL-4 mRNA upon concanavalin A-induced liver injury (El-Karef et al., 2007). Furthermore, tenascin-C may be involved in lymphocyte activation although both stimulatory and inhibitory effects have been reported. Tenascin-C significantly stimulates the secretion of IL-5, IL-13, IFN-g and immunoglobulin-E from spleen lymphocytes (Nakahara et al., 2006). However, it has inhibitory effect on the anti CD3-induced activation of human peripheral blood T cells irrespectively of costimulatory molecules used (Hemesath et al., 1994; Hibino et al, 1998) and it was also found to inhibit T cell activation induced by alloantigens (Ruegg et al., 1989).

Conversely, Tenascin-C synthesis is a target of inflammatory stimuli: it is specifically induced in immune myeloid cells by ligands to TLRs located at the cell surface (TLR2, 4, and 5), but not by those targeting TLRs in the endosome; (TLR3 or TLR8) (Goh et al., 2010). Tenascin-C expression is rapidly and transiently induced in immune myeloid cells in response to tissue injury and infection (Midwood & Orend, 2009). It therefore appears that induction of tenascin-C in an inflammatory setting would drive TLR4 activation leading to synthesis of more tenascin-C, perhaps resulting in a nonresolving loop of chronic inflammation (Goh et al., 2010).

3.4 Matricellular protein's role in the TGF-β signaling pathway

TGF-β is pivotal in TV and in fibrosis in general. Several matricellular proteins are involved in promoting TGF signalling. They are either involved in promoting synthesis of TGF (osteonectin, periostin), activating of the cytokine itself (thrombospondin-1 and possibly periostin) or enhancing the signalling of its receptor (osteonectin). In addition, some matricellular proteins are downstream targets of TGF signalling (CCN2). To enhance understanding of the different modes of action it is necessary to explain the complex pathway of TGF activation: Precursors of the TGF-β isoforms 1 to 3 are cleaved by a furin protease to generate mature TGF-β and its propeptide, also known as latency-associated peptide (LAP). LAP and mature TGF-β remain noncovalently associated in a complex called the small latency complex (SLC), and in this form, TGF-β remains inactive. The LAPs then binds to one of the latent TGF-β–binding proteins (LTBPs) to form large latent complexes (LLCs). The LTBPs bind to ECM proteins including fibrillins and fibronectin, thereby incorporating the different latent TGF-β isoforms into extracellular matrices. There are several mechanisms for activation, one of them involving thrombospondin-1 binding and LAP dissociation (Hynes, 2009).

Thrombospondin-1-induced activation of TGF-β was reported for first time in 1992 by Murphy-Ullrich and coworkers (Murphy-Ullrich et al., 1992) and since then thrombospondin-1 domains responsible for TGF binding have been identified (reviewed H. Chen, Herndon, & Lawler, 2000). The significance of this process confirmed both in vitro and in vivo, including angiotensin II–induced upregulation of thrombospondin leading to TGF-β activation by cardiac and renal cells (Zhou et al., 2006) as well as a role for thrombospondin-1 in mesangial proliferative glomerulonephritis (Daniel et al., 2004) and diabetic nephropathy (Daniel et al., 2007).

Osteonectin/SPARC acts at two levels: first, it is involved in stimulating TGF production (Schiemann et al., 2003) and second, osteonectin modulates the TGF-β1-dependent phosphorylation of Smad-2 in primary mesangial cells through an interaction with the TGF-β1-receptor complex, but only in the presence of TGF-β1 bound to its cognate type II receptor (Francki et al., 2004). Osteonectin mediated modulation TGF-β signaling has been also shown in cardiac fibroblasts in vitro. Most importantly, infusion of TGF-β can rescue the cardiac rupture phenotype in osteonectin-null mice (Schellings et al., 2009).

In a recently published study Sidhu and coworkers demonstrated increased TGF-β production and enhanced TGF-β bioactivity both in periostin-overexpressing epithelial cells and in primary airway epithelial cells stimulated with recombinant periostin and suggested that periostin is an upstream regulator of TGF-β activation in a mechanism involving MMP2 and -9 (Sidhu et al., 2010). On the other hand, CCN2/CTGF acts as a downstream mediator of TGF-β-induced fibroblasts proliferation, myofibroblast differentiation (Grotendorst et al., 2004; Kothapalli et al., 1997) and collagen synthesis (Duncan et al., 1999). CTGF synthesis is induced by TGF-β in fibroblasts via a unique TGF-β response element in the CTGF promoter, and blockade of CTGF synthesis or action effectively inhibits these TGF-β effects on fibroblasts. Further research has revealed that the two domains of CTGF function mediate two distinct biological effects, the N-terminal domain myofibroblast differentiation and collagen synthesis and the C-terminal domain fibroblast proliferation (Grotendorst & Duncan, 2005). Interestingly, another member of CCN family - CCN3 (Nov) may act as an endogenous negative regulator of CCN2 with the capacity to limit the overproduction of extracellular matrix (ECM), and thus prevent or ameliorate fibrosis (Riser et al., 2010). Over-expression of the CCN3 gene in mesangial cells markedly down-regulates CCN2 activity and blocks ECM over-accumulation stimulated by TGF-β1. Conversely, TGF-β1 treatment reduces endogenous CCN3 expression and increases CCN2 activity and matrix accumulation (Riser et al., 2010). Additionally, when cultured mesangial cells are exposed to exogenous CCN3 protein, TGF-β stimulated increase in CCN2 is attenuated in a dose-dependent manner (Riser et al., 2009).

Osteopontin, similar to CCN2, also mediates the TGF-β signaling involved in the differentiation of fibroblasts into myofibroblasts. This conclusion is based on the observation that α-smooth muscle actin is not expressed in TGF-β–treated cardiac fibroblasts isolated from osteopontin-null mice and additionally confirmed by small interfering RNA knockdown of osteopontin in fibroblasts from wild-type mice (Lenga et al., 2008).

3.5 Matricellular proteins in myofibroblast differentiation and SMC recruitment

TGF-β is thought to provide a crucial signal that initiates differentiation of myofibroblasts (Leask, 2010), partly acting by altering focal adhesion kinase activatity, up-regulating expression of integrin receptors and induction of the fibronectin splice variant ectodomain (ED)-A (Ffrench-Constant et al., 1989; Serini et al., 1998). While matricelular proteins can influence myofibroblast differentiation via modulation of TGF-β signalling as described in previous section, there is growing evidence that matricellular proteins can influence fibroblast recruitment and differentiation also by other mechanisms.

3.5.1 Tenascin C

Tamaoki and coworkers, studying tissue repair after myocardial injury observed that the appearance of myofibroblasts was delayed in tenascin-C KO mice, although myocardial repair appeared to proceed normally. Moreover, cardiac fibroblasts from tenascin-C KO mice showed lower cell migration and α-SMA expression than WT cells that synthesize tenascin-C in culture. Addition of tenascin-C to tenascin-C-null cells recovered both cell migration and α-SMA expression. Functional domains of tenascin-C protein responsible for inducing myofibroblast differentiation were mapped to alternatively spliced FNIII repeats (but not the conserved repeats) and the FGB domain. In contrast, the molecular signal that promoted migration of cardiac fibroblasts was mapped to the domain of conserved FNIII repeats and the FGB domain (Tamaoki et al., 2005).

3.5.2 Periostin

Recently, Shimazaki and coworkers reported that impaired cardiac healing after an acute myocardial infarction in periostin-KO mice was associated with reduced numbers of alpha smooth muscle actin-positive cells. The authors suggested a model in which periostin signals via αv-integrin, FAK, and Akt, activates cell migration of cardiac fibroblasts from outside into the infarct region, and then supports their differentiation into αSMA-positive fibroblasts, resulting in enhanced stiffness of the LV wall through collagen synthesis after AMI (Shimazaki et al., 2008). Interestingly, periostin has been shown also to mediate vascular smooth muscle cell migration through mechanisms similar to those described above engaging the integrins αvβ3 and αvβ5 and focal adhesion kinase (FAK) pathway (Li et al., 2010).

3.6 Matricellular proteins in ECM assembly and collagen fibrillogenesis

An identification of the factors that control collagen fibril formation and ECM assembly is critical for an understanding of tissue organization and the mechanisms that lead to fibrosis. There is growing evidence that matricellular proteins may play an important role in these processes not only via effects on TGF-β signaling pathway. Below we have listed a few examples suggesting potential mechanisms of matricellular proteins involvement in collagen synthesis and maturation.

3.6.1 Tenascin X – effect on matrix mechanical properties

A crucial role in tenascin-X collagen biology is suggested by the fact that its deficiency is associated with the Ehlers-Danlos Syndrome in humans (Burch et al., 1997). Major clinical symptoms consist of skin hyperextensibility and joint laxity, while ultrastructural analyses reveal abnormalities in collagen fibril networks and elastic fibre morphology. Mice deficient in tenascin-X partly reproduced this phenotype (Mao et al., 2002). In vitro studies revealed that tenascin-X interacts with fibrillar collagen type I, III and V when they are in native conformation. Additional studies indicated that both epidermal growth factor repeats and the fibrinogen-like domain are involved in this interaction (Lethias et al., 2006) and although the presence of tenascin-X does not significantly influence the main parameters of fibrillogenesis and diameter of fibrils, mechanical analysis of collagen gels showed an increased compressive resistance of the gels containing tenascin-X, indicating that this protein might be directly involved in determining the mechanical properties of collagen-rich tissues in vivo (Margaron et al., 2010).

3.6.2 Osteonectin – effect on procollagen I processing

Adult osteonectin-null mice exhibit decreased amounts of collagen in skin (Bradshaw et al., 2003). In addition, fibrotic deposition of collagen in mice with bleomycin-induced pulmonary fibrosis is diminished in the absence of osteonectin (Strandjord et al., 1999), Moreover, Rentz and coworkers investigated collagen I production in osteonectin-null dermal fibroblasts observing that osteonectin might be involved in regulation of procollagen I processing (Rentz et al., 2007). The α1(I) and α2(I) subunits of procollagen I are synthesized with N- and C-propeptides that are enzymatically released by specific proteases. Processing of procollagen I to collagen I is essential for correct assembly of collagen fibrils and regulation of procollagen processing has been proposed as a potential regulatory event in collagen fibril assembly (Prockop & Kivirikko, 1995). Although osteonectin-null dermal fibroblasts exhibited an increased association of collagen I with cell layers and enhanced processing of procollagen1(I) to collagen1(I). The processed collagen I was not efficiently incorporated into osteonectin-null detergent-insoluble cell layers, and collagen fibers that formed on osteonectin-null cells did not persist to the same extent as those on WT cells (Rentz et al., 2007).

3.6.3 Periostin – an effect on collagen I cross-linking

Collagen fibrils from periostin-deficient mice show reduced size, organisation, and less efficient cross-linking (Norris et al., 2007; Shimazaki et al., 2008). Recently, Maruhashi and coworkers (Maruhashi et al., 2010) proposed a model to explain periostin's role in determining ECM integrity. Collagen fibrils are stabilized by the formation of intra- and intermolecular cross-linking that is catalyzed by the enzyme lysyl oxidase (LOX). The activity of LOX is regulated by proteolytic cleavage of its inactive precursor, pro-LOX, by BMP-1 (bone morphogenetic protein-1; also known as pro-collagen C-proteinase) (Uzel et al., 2001). Periostin binds to BMP-1 and promotes the proteolytic activation of pro-LOX. As it has been shown that periostin also interacts with fibronectin (Takayama et al., 2006), the model suggest periostin-mediated scaffolding for the interaction between pro-LOX and BMP-1 on the fibronectin matrix (Maruhashi et al., 2010).

4. Matricellular proteins in therapy

Although modulation of matricellular protein function has not yet been subject to clinical trials, there is growing evidence from experiments in animal models that this approach can be beneficial in many diseases including fibrosis. Here, we present a few of models of experimental therapy involving matricellular proteins.

4.1 Depletion of microcellular protein by antisense or siRNA

Adenovirus-mediated inhibition of osteonectin markedly attenuated the development of hepatic fibrosis in rats treated with thioacetamide, as assessed by decreased collagen deposition, lower hepatic content of hydroxyproline and less advanced morphometric stage of fibrosis. Osteonectin depletion also reduced inflammatory activity and suppressed transdifferentiation of hepatic stellate cell to the myofibroblasts-like phenotype (Camino et al., 2008). In another approach, osteonectin siRNA treatment through subcutaneous injection or intratracheal instillation was found to markedly reduce fibrotic changes in skin and lungs in murine models of skin and lung fibrosis induced by bleomycin (Wang et al., 2010).

Morover, antisense oligonucleotides against thrombospondin-1 were used to inhibit activation of TGF-β in a rat model of mesangial proliferative glomerulonephritis, in which

TGF-β has been demonstrated to mediate renal fibrosis. The antisense-mediated reduction of thrombospondin did not reduce the expression of TGF-β but rather inhibited the TGF-β-dependent smad-signalling pathway, as well as the transcription of TGF-beta target genes, resulting in a markedly suppressed accumulation of extracellular matrix (Daniel et al., 2003).

4.2 Modification of matricellular protein function by antagonist

In a rat model of type 1 diabetes in which diabetic cardiomyopathy is exacerbated by abdominal aortic coarctation, Belmadani and coworkers observed that a peptide antagonist of thrombospondin-1-dependent TGF-β activation prevented progression of cardiac fibrosis and improved cardiac function (Belmadani et al., 2007). In an analogous experiment, treatment with a peptide antagonist of thrombospondin-1 attenuated renal interstitial fibrosis in rats with unilateral ureteral obstruction (Xie et al., 2010).

4.3 Overexpression of matricellular protein

Thrombospondin-2 overexpression via thigh muscle transfection was studied in the anti-Thy1 glomerulonephritis model. Muscular overexpression of thrombospondin-2 reduced glomerular TGF-β activation and glomerular extracellular matrix formation as determined by collagen IV and fibronectin. In addition, activation of mesangial cells to the myofibroblast-like phenotype was also significantly decreased in thrombospondin-2-overexpressing animals (Daniel, Wagner, Hohenstein, & Hugo, 2009). Additionally, thrombospondin 1 overexpression was suggested as a gene therapeutic strategy in collagen-induced arthritis (CIA). Direct intraarticular administration of adenoviral vectors encoding thrombospondin-1 significantly ameliorated the clinical course of CIA in rat model (Jou et al., 2005).

5. Models of fibrosis

Animal models of chronic allograft injury have been comprehensively described in a recent review (Bedi et al., 2010).

5.1 Heterotopic cardiac transplantation

The model of heterotopic cardiac transplantation is and has been widely used to study chronic allograft injury and rejection. It also provides information relevant to graft ischemia-reperfusion injury, allorejection and immunosuppressants, as well as physiologic changes that take place post-transplant in vascularized organs. In comparison to orthotopic transplantation, the heterotopic procedure is technically less demanding and does not require a cardiopulmonary bypass. After pioneer transplantation experiments in large animals, Abbott et al. described a method of vascularised abdominal heterotopic heart transplantation in rats in 1964 (Abbott et al., 1964). Ono and Lindsay improved the technique by end-to-side anastomosis of the donor vessels to the recipient's aorta and IVC, resulting in a higher recipient survival rate (Ono & Lindsey, 1969). This method has been widely used, adopted to use in mice and improved by several modifications (Hasegawa et al., 2007; Shan et al., 2010).

Of particular relevance to TV, Adams et al. described cardiac allografting across minor histocompatibility barriers (Lewis-F344 model) (Adams et al., 1993). Advantages of the

Lewis-F344 model are commercial availability and easily recognizable inflammatory stages of lesion development. On the other hand, grafts have relatively low long-term survival rates (25%) and they show substantially more severe mononuclear infiltration and necrosis when compared to human TV lesions (Adams et al., 1993), unless they were exposed to high levels of cyclosporin, in which case TV failed to develop (Poston et al., 1999). Although the Lewis-F344 model remains commonly used, Poston et al. argued that a model in which TV developed despite immunosuppression, would more appropriately reflect a situation where cell mediated alloimmunity is not the sole or major pathogenesis (Poston et al., 1999). This situation is seen in the PVG (Piebald Viral Glaxo, RT1c)-to-ACI (August Copenhagen Irish, RT1a) which is a fully-mismatched MHC class II model. However, a disadvantage of the PVG-to-ACI model is that it fails to induce myocardial rejection. Nevertheless, in this model, rapamycin, but not cyclosporin, is capable of reducing the degree of chronic graft vascular disease and opens the door for investigators to study chronic injury in a model that is relatively resistant to T-cell– directed immunosuppressants (like cyclosporin) but susceptible to novel agents whose mechanism of actions lies beyond reduction in T-cell–mediated immunity.

Murine models of chronic allograft injury include those involving different strains with minor histoincompatibilities, which usually leads to a smoldering immunologic response within the allograft and ultimately, chronic injury (Bedi et al., 2010).

An established mouse model of TV is an MHC class II-mismatched heterotopic graft from B6.C.H-2-bm12 (bm12) into a wild-type C57BL/6 (B6, H-2b) mouse. Bm12 mice are a variant strain of C57BL/6 mice, in which a spontaneous mutation has occurred in the I-Ab locus, designated I-Abm12. In this single MHC class II mismatch model, the majority of bm12 cardiac allografts survive up to 100 days and develop significant vasculopathy, notable for intraluminal accumulation of mononuclear leukocytes (at 4 weeks posttransplant), intimal lesions (by 8 weeks), and accumulation of smooth muscle cells signifying fibroproliferative arteriosclerotic lesions (by 12 weeks; Fig. 2). The limited alloreactive T-cell activation and emergence of a population of regulatory T cells allow long-term allograft survival with the development of significant vasculopathy (Bedi et al., 2010).

As in rat models, heterotopic cardiac transplantation between fully MHC-mismatched mouse strains has been described as models for studying chronic rejection with the use of postoperative immunosuppressants to prevent acute rejection. In one model, anti-CD40L is administered after B6-to- BALB/c (H2d) heterotopic cardiac transplantation. Without manipulation, cardiac allografts are promptly rejected; however, if treated with anti-CD40L, acute rejection is ameliorated, and recipients develop chronic rejection. In this model, approximately 50% of cardiac allografts survive 100 days, but with severe evidence of histologic chronic allograft changes (Bedi et al., 2010).

5.2 Aorta transplantation

Abdominal aorta transplantation has been widely used in rodents as a model for TV (i.e. Murphy, Bicknell, & Nicholson, 2003)) and involves substitution of a part of the recipient's distal aorta with a donor graft. One of the first aortic allograft models for chronic rejection in the rat was described by Mennader (Mennander et al., 1991) and Isik (Isik et al., 1992). They revealed histologic features that parallel those seen in the vessels of human transplanted organs (Isik et al., 1992). Similar methods in mice have been described by Koulack et al. (Koulack et al., 1995) and have been further modified (i.e. (Ensminger et al., 2002)). The histologic features are an initial increase in mononuclear inflammatory cells with gradually increasing numbers of smooth muscle cells resulting in intimal thickening of the aorta and at later time points in deposition of extracellular matrix and collagen fibrils (Isik et al., 1992).

Aortic allografts transplantation represents an alternative model for evaluation of the influence of novel transplant strategies on transplant arteriosclerosis. Vascular changes can be easily and more precisely quantified due to faciliated access to the aortic graft thus providing representative sections (Isik et al., 1992; Mennander et al., 1991). In contrast, quantification of TV in rat and mouse cardiac allografts is reportedly difficult and the interpretation of the data obtained controversial (Ensminger et al., 2000; Isik et al., 1992).

The aortic transplantation is a useful model for the study of vascular repair. Due to the absence of the impact of supporting parenchyma it is questionable whether vascular changes in aortic allografts are representative for chronic vascular rejection in solid-organ transplants (Libby & Pober, 2001). Nevertheless, Ensminger et al. reported in a combined cardiac and aortic transplant model on equivalent outcome of TV in abdominal aortic allografts in the presence as well as in the absence of an additional organ transplant (Ensminger et al., 2000). Moreover, although heterotopic cardiac transplantation might be a more suitable model, the aortic transplantation model is helpful in understanding the endothelial milieu during chronic allograft injury.

5.3 Other models of cardiac fibrosis

Most other models of cardiac fibrosis involve mechanic or pharmacologic intervention aimed at increasing the cardiac workload. The mechanic approach involves partial constriction at various levels of the aortic arch. The pharmacologic approach involves the infusion of angiotensin or aldosterone. Angiotensin treatment leads to fibrosis development within 2 weeks and increases with time (Sun & Weber, 2005), whereas the aldosterone model also requires reduction of functional kidney mass (unilateral nephrectomy) and subsequent high sodium diet, therefore requiring more than 4 weeks to develop fibrosis (Sun & Weber, 2005).

5.4 Selected features of non-cardiac models of fibrosis

A large number of fibrosis models in other organs have been described and are thought to have particular relevance to fibrosis in that specific organ. Inducing agents can be alloreactivity, chemical irritants, high-fat diet (relevant to liver fibrosis) or secretory obstruction (bile or urine). However, it is worth noting that a comparison between organs may provide a more efficient search for core pathways essential to convert an initial stimulus to the development of fibrosis (Mehal et al., 2011). Likewise, none of the models, currently considered relevant to understanding cardiac fibrosis development, are well suited for "high-throughput" analyses because they are technically demanding and require a relatively long time to develop the lesion.

Unilateral ureteral obstruction (UUO) is an inducible animal model in rodents for human obstructive nephropathy leading to tubolointerstitial fibrosis. It has become a standard model of nonimmunological tubulointerstitial fibrosis in which the ureter of one kidney is obstructed by ligation. Obstruction can be partial or total. With complete obstruction, fibrosis can generally be observed within 1-2 weeks, depending on the species and strain used in the experimental setting. A substantial advantage of the UUO model over complex transplantation models is technical simplicity and a relatively short time required to develop the lesions. Other assets are absence of exogenous toxin and the contralateral organ serving as control (Chevalier et al., 2009).

6. Conclusion

Transplant vasculopathy and interstitial fibrosis remain key clinical obstacles to achieve long-term survival of solid organ allografts. Although to date relatively little data has been generated to address the role of matricellular proteins directly in this context, there is considerable circumstantial evidence from surrounding fields to foresee that their functions may be central to allograft-associated fibrosis development. Several models of cardiac fibrosis are well-established but time consuming. This limitation may be seen in light of the recently proposed strategy to identify core pathways of fibrosis by simultaneously comparing the process in several different organs.

7. References

Abbott, C. P., Lindsey, E. S., Creech, O., Jr., & Dewitt, C. W. (1964). A Technique for Heart Transplantation in the Rat. *Arch Surg, 89*, 645-652.

Adams, D. H., Russell, M. E., Hancock, W. W., Sayegh, M. H., Wyner, L. R., & Karnovsky, M. J. (1993). Chronic rejection in experimental cardiac transplantation: studies in the Lewis-F344 model. *Immunol Rev, 134*, 5-19.

Adams, J. C., & Lawler, J. (2004). The thrombospondins. *Int J Biochem Cell Biol, 36*(6), 961-968.

Ashkar, S., Weber, G. F., Panoutsakopoulou, V., Sanchirico, M. E., Jansson, M., Zawaideh, S., et al. (2000). Eta-1 (osteopontin): an early component of type-1 (cell-mediated) immunity. *Science, 287*(5454), 860-864.

Bedi, D. S., Riella, L. V., Tullius, S. G., & Chandraker, A. (2010). Animal models of chronic allograft injury: contributions and limitations to understanding the mechanism of long-term graft dysfunction. *Transplantation, 90*(9), 935-944.

Belmadani, S., Bernal, J., Wei, C. C., Pallero, M. A., Dell'italia, L., Murphy-Ullrich, J. E., et al. (2007). A thrombospondin-1 antagonist of transforming growth factor-beta activation blocks cardiomyopathy in rats with diabetes and elevated angiotensin II. *Am J Pathol, 171*(3), 777-789.

Bornstein, P. (1995). Diversity of function is inherent in matricellular proteins: an appraisal of thrombospondin 1. *J Cell Biol, 130*(3), 503-506.

Bornstein, P., & Sage, E. H. (2002). Matricellular proteins: extracellular modulators of cell function. *Curr Opin Cell Biol, 14*(5), 608-616.

Bradshaw, A. D., Puolakkainen, P., Dasgupta, J., Davidson, J. M., Wight, T. N., & Helene Sage, E. (2003). SPARC-null mice display abnormalities in the dermis characterized by decreased collagen fibril diameter and reduced tensile strength. *J Invest Dermatol, 120*(6), 949-955.

Brekken, R. A., & Sage, E. H. (2000). SPARC, a matricellular protein: at the crossroads of cell-matrix. *Matrix Biol, 19*(7), 569-580.

Bruemmer, D., Collins, A. R., Noh, G., Wang, W., Territo, M., Arias-Magallona, S., et al. (2003). Angiotensin II-accelerated atherosclerosis and aneurysm formation is attenuated in osteopontin-deficient mice. *J Clin Invest, 112*(9), 1318-1331.

Burch, G. H., Gong, Y., Liu, W., Dettman, R. W., Curry, C. J., Smith, L., et al. (1997). Tenascin-X deficiency is associated with Ehlers-Danlos syndrome. *Nat Genet, 17*(1), 104-108.

Camino, A. M., Atorrasagasti, C., Maccio, D., Prada, F., Salvatierra, E., Rizzo, M., et al. (2008). Adenovirus-mediated inhibition of SPARC attenuates liver fibrosis in rats. *J Gene Med, 10*(9), 993-1004.

Chen, C. C., & Lau, L. F. (2009). Functions and mechanisms of action of CCN matricellular proteins. *Int J Biochem Cell Biol, 41*(4), 771-783.

Chen, H., Herndon, M. E., & Lawler, J. (2000). The cell biology of thrombospondin-1. *Matrix Biol, 19*(7), 597-614.

Chevalier, R. L., Forbes, M. S., & Thornhill, B. A. (2009). Ureteral obstruction as a model of renal interstitial fibrosis and obstructive nephropathy. *Kidney Int, 75*(11), 1145-1152.

Chiquet-Ehrismann, R., & Chiquet, M. (2003). Tenascins: regulation and putative functions during pathological stress. *J Pathol, 200*(4), 488-499.

Clark, R. A., Erickson, H. P., & Springer, T. A. (1997). Tenascin supports lymphocyte rolling. *J Cell Biol, 137*(3), 755-765.

Conway, S. J., & Molkentin, J. D. (2008). Periostin as a heterofunctional regulator of cardiac development and disease. *Curr Genomics, 9*(8), 548-555.

Cox, T. R., & Erler, J. T. (2011). Remodeling and homeostasis of the extracellular matrix: implications for fibrotic diseases and cancer. *Dis Model Mech, 4*(2), 165-178.

Daniel, C., Schaub, K., Amann, K., Lawler, J., & Hugo, C. (2007). Thrombospondin-1 is an endogenous activator of TGF-beta in experimental diabetic nephropathy in vivo. *Diabetes, 56*(12), 2982-2989.

Daniel, C., Takabatake, Y., Mizui, M., Isaka, Y., Kawashi, H., Rupprecht, H., et al. (2003). Antisense oligonucleotides against thrombospondin-1 inhibit activation of tgf-beta in fibrotic renal disease in the rat in vivo. *Am J Pathol, 163*(3), 1185-1192.

Daniel, C., Wagner, A., Hohenstein, B., & Hugo, C. (2009). Thrombospondin-2 therapy ameliorates experimental glomerulonephritis via inhibition of cell proliferation, inflammation, and TGF-beta activation. *Am J Physiol Renal Physiol, 297*(5), F1299-1309.

Daniel, C., Wiede, J., Krutzsch, H. C., Ribeiro, S. M., Roberts, D. D., Murphy-Ullrich, J. E., et al. (2004). Thrombospondin-1 is a major activator of TGF-beta in fibrotic renal disease in the rat in vivo. *Kidney Int, 65*(2), 459-468.

Duncan, M. R., Frazier, K. S., Abramson, S., Williams, S., Klapper, H., Huang, X., et al. (1999). Connective tissue growth factor mediates transforming growth factor beta-induced collagen synthesis: down-regulation by cAMP. *Faseb J, 13*(13), 1774-1786.

El-Karef, A., Yoshida, T., Gabazza, E. C., Nishioka, T., Inada, H., Sakakura, T., et al. (2007). Deficiency of tenascin-C attenuates liver fibrosis in immune-mediated chronic hepatitis in mice. *J Pathol, 211*(1), 86-94.

Elefteriou, F., Exposito, J. Y., Garrone, R., & Lethias, C. (1999). Cell adhesion to tenascin-X mapping of cell adhesion sites and identification of integrin receptors. *Eur J Biochem, 263*(3), 840-848.

Ellison, J. A., Velier, J. J., Spera, P., Jonak, Z. L., Wang, X., Barone, F. C., et al. (1998). Osteopontin and its integrin receptor alpha(v)beta3 are upregulated during formation of the glial scar after focal stroke. *Stroke, 29*(8), 1698-1706; discussion 1707.

Ensminger, S. M., Billing, J. S., Morris, P. J., & Wood, K. J. (2000). Development of a combined cardiac and aortic transplant model to investigate the development of transplant arteriosclerosis in the mouse. *J Heart Lung Transplant, 19*(11), 1039-1046.

Ensminger, S. M., Spriewald, B. M., Witzke, O., Morrison, K., Pajaro, O. E., Morris, P. J., et al. (2002). Kinetics of transplant arteriosclerosis in MHC-Class I mismatched and fully allogeneic mouse aortic allografts. *Transplantation, 73*(7), 1068-1074.

Ffrench-Constant, C., Van de Water, L., Dvorak, H. F., & Hynes, R. O. (1989). Reappearance of an embryonic pattern of fibronectin splicing during wound healing in the adult rat. *J Cell Biol, 109*(2), 903-914.

Fischer, J. W. (2007). Tenascin-C: a key molecule in graft stenosis. *Cardiovasc Res, 74*(3), 335-336.

Francki, A., McClure, T. D., Brekken, R. A., Motamed, K., Murri, C., Wang, T., et al. (2004). SPARC regulates TGF-beta1-dependent signaling in primary glomerular mesangial cells. *J Cell Biochem, 91*(5), 915-925.

Frangogiannis, N. G., Ren, G., Dewald, O., Zymek, P., Haudek, S., Koerting, A., et al. (2005). Critical role of endogenous thrombospondin-1 in preventing expansion of healing myocardial infarcts. *Circulation, 111*(22), 2935-2942.

Franz, M., Grun, K., Richter, P., Brehm, B. R., Fritzenwanger, M., Hekmat, K., et al. (2010). Extra cellular matrix remodelling after heterotopic rat heart transplantation: gene expression profiling and involvement of ED-A+ fibronectin, alpha-smooth muscle actin and B+ tenascin-C in chronic cardiac allograft rejection. *Histochem Cell Biol, 134*(5), 503-517.

Gamba, A., Mammana, C., Fiocchi, R., Iamele, L., & Mamprin, F. (2000). Cyclosporine and graft coronary artery disease after heart transplantation. *Compr Ther, 26*(2), 121-126.

Geffrotin, C., Garrido, J. J., Tremet, L., & Vaiman, M. (1995). Distinct tissue distribution in pigs of tenascin-X and tenascin-C transcripts. *Eur J Biochem, 231*(1), 83-92.

Giachelli, C. M., Bae, N., Almeida, M., Denhardt, D. T., Alpers, C. E., & Schwartz, S. M. (1993). Osteopontin is elevated during neointima formation in rat arteries and is a novel component of human atherosclerotic plaques. *J Clin Invest, 92*(4), 1686-1696.

Giachelli, C. M., Lombardi, D., Johnson, R. J., Murry, C. E., & Almeida, M. (1998). Evidence for a role of osteopontin in macrophage infiltration in response to pathological stimuli in vivo. *Am J Pathol, 152*(2), 353-358.

Goh, F. G., Piccinini, A. M., Krausgruber, T., Udalova, I. A., & Midwood, K. S. (2010). Transcriptional regulation of the endogenous danger signal tenascin-C: a novel autocrine loop in inflammation. *J Immunol, 184*(5), 2655-2662.

Greenwood, J. A., & Murphy-Ullrich, J. E. (1998). Signaling of de-adhesion in cellular regulation and motility. *Microsc Res Tech, 43*(5), 420-432.

Grotendorst, G. R., & Duncan, M. R. (2005). Individual domains of connective tissue growth factor regulate fibroblast proliferation and myofibroblast differentiation. *Faseb J, 19*(7), 729-738.

Grotendorst, G. R., Rahmanie, H., & Duncan, M. R. (2004). Combinatorial signaling pathways determine fibroblast proliferation and myofibroblast differentiation. *Faseb J, 18*(3), 469-479.

Hasegawa, T., Visovatti, S. H., Hyman, M. C., Hayasaki, T., & Pinsky, D. J. (2007). Heterotopic vascularized murine cardiac transplantation to study graft arteriopathy. *Nat Protoc, 2*(3), 471-480.

Hemesath, T. J., Marton, L. S., & Stefansson, K. (1994). Inhibition of T cell activation by the extracellular matrix protein tenascin. *J Immunol, 152*(11), 5199-5207.

Hibino, S., Kato, K., Kudoh, S., Yagita, H., & Okumura, K. (1998). Tenascin suppresses CD3-mediated T cell activation. *Biochem Biophys Res Commun, 250*(1), 119-124.

Hinz, B. (2010). The myofibroblast: paradigm for a mechanically active cell. *J Biomech, 43*(1), 146-155.

Hynes, R. O. (2009). The extracellular matrix: not just pretty fibrils. *Science, 326*(5957), 1216-1219.

Imanaka-Yoshida, K., Hiroe, M., Nishikawa, T., Ishiyama, S., Shimojo, T., Ohta, Y., et al. (2001). Tenascin-C modulates adhesion of cardiomyocytes to extracellular matrix during tissue remodeling after myocardial infarction. *Lab Invest, 81*(7), 1015-1024.

Imanaka-Yoshida, K., Hiroe, M., Yasutomi, Y., Toyozaki, T., Tsuchiya, T., Noda, N., et al. (2002). Tenascin-C is a useful marker for disease activity in myocarditis. *J Pathol, 197*(3), 388-394.

Isik, F. F., McDonald, T. O., Ferguson, M., Yamanaka, E., & Gordon, D. (1992). Transplant arteriosclerosis in a rat aortic model. *Am J Pathol, 141*(5), 1139-1149.

Jou, I. M., Shiau, A. L., Chen, S. Y., Wang, C. R., Shieh, D. B., Tsai, C. S., et al. (2005). Thrombospondin 1 as an effective gene therapeutic strategy in collagen-induced arthritis. *Arthritis Rheum, 52*(1), 339-344.

Kanayama, M., Kurotaki, D., Morimoto, J., Asano, T., Matsui, Y., Nakayama, Y., et al. (2009). Alpha9 integrin and its ligands constitute critical joint microenvironments for development of autoimmune arthritis. *J Immunol, 182*(12), 8015-8025.

Khanna, A. (2005). Tacrolimus and cyclosporinein vitro and in vivo induce osteopontin mRNA and protein expression in renal tissues. *Nephron Exp Nephrol, 101*(4), e119-126.

Kii, I., Nishiyama, T., Li, M., Matsumoto, K., Saito, M., Amizuka, N., et al. (2010). Incorporation of tenascin-C into the extracellular matrix by periostin underlies an extracellular meshwork architecture. *J Biol Chem, 285*(3), 2028-2039.

Koh, A., da Silva, A. P., Bansal, A. K., Bansal, M., Sun, C., Lee, H., et al. (2007). Role of osteopontin in neutrophil function. *Immunology, 122*(4), 466-475.

Komatsubara, I., Murakami, T., Kusachi, S., Nakamura, K., Hirohata, S., Hayashi, J., et al. (2003). Spatially and temporally different expression of osteonectin and osteopontin in the infarct zone of experimentally induced myocardial infarction in rats. *Cardiovasc Pathol, 12*(4), 186-194.

Kothapalli, D., Frazier, K. S., Welply, A., Segarini, P. R., & Grotendorst, G. R. (1997). Transforming growth factor beta induces anchorage-independent growth of NRK fibroblasts via a connective tissue growth factor-dependent signaling pathway. *Cell Growth Differ, 8*(1), 61-68.

Koulack, J., McAlister, V. C., Giacomantonio, C. A., Bitter-Suermann, H., MacDonald, A. S., & Lee, T. D. (1995). Development of a mouse aortic transplant model of chronic rejection. *Microsurgery, 16*(2), 110-113.

Krishnamurthy, P., Peterson, J. T., Subramanian, V., Singh, M., & Singh, K. (2009). Inhibition of matrix metalloproteinases improves left ventricular function in mice lacking osteopontin after myocardial infarction. *Mol Cell Biochem, 322*(1-2), 53-62.

Kruzynska-Frejtag, A., Machnicki, M., Rogers, R., Markwald, R. R., & Conway, S. J. (2001). Periostin (an osteoblast-specific factor) is expressed within the embryonic mouse heart during valve formation. *Mech Dev, 103*(1-2), 183-188.

Kular, L., Pakradouni, J., Kitabgi, P., Laurent, M., & Martinerie, C. (2011). The CCN family: a new class of inflammation modulators? *Biochimie, 93*(3), 377-388.

Leask, A. (2010). Potential therapeutic targets for cardiac fibrosis: TGFbeta, angiotensin, endothelin, CCN2, and PDGF, partners in fibroblast activation. *Circ Res, 106*(11), 1675-1680.

Lenga, Y., Koh, A., Perera, A. S., McCulloch, C. A., Sodek, J., & Zohar, R. (2008). Osteopontin expression is required for myofibroblast differentiation. *Circ Res, 102*(3), 319-327.

Lethias, C., Carisey, A., Comte, J., Cluzel, C., & Exposito, J. Y. (2006). A model of tenascin-X integration within the collagenous network. *FEBS Lett, 580*(26), 6281-6285.

Li, G., Jin, R., Norris, R. A., Zhang, L., Yu, S., Wu, F., et al. (2010). Periostin mediates vascular smooth muscle cell migration through the integrins alphavbeta3 and alphavbeta5 and focal adhesion kinase (FAK) pathway. *Atherosclerosis, 208*(2), 358-365.

Libby, P., & Pober, J. S. (2001). Chronic rejection. *Immunity, 14*(4), 387-397.

Lund, S. A., Giachelli, C. M., & Scatena, M. (2009). The role of osteopontin in inflammatory processes. *J Cell Commun Signal, 3*(3-4), 311-322.

Mao, J. R., Taylor, G., Dean, W. B., Wagner, D. R., Afzal, V., Lotz, J. C., et al. (2002). Tenascin-X deficiency mimics Ehlers-Danlos syndrome in mice through alteration of collagen deposition. *Nat Genet, 30*(4), 421-425.

Margaron, Y., Bostan, L., Exposito, J. Y., Malbouyres, M., Trunfio-Sfarghiu, A. M., Berthier, Y., et al. (2010). Tenascin-X increases the stiffness of collagen gels without affecting fibrillogenesis. *Biophys Chem, 147*(1-2), 87-91.

Maruhashi, T., Kii, I., Saito, M., & Kudo, A. (2010). Interaction between periostin and BMP-1 promotes proteolytic activation of lysyl oxidase. *J Biol Chem, 285*(17), 13294-13303.

Matsui, Y., Morimoto, J., & Uede, T. (2010). Role of matricellular proteins in cardiac tissue remodeling after myocardial infarction. *World J Biol Chem, 1*(5), 69-80.

Mehal, W. Z., Iredale, J., & Friedman, S. L. (2011). Scraping fibrosis: expressway to the core of fibrosis. *Nat Med, 17*(5), 552-553.

Mennander, A., Tiisala, S., Halttunen, J., Yilmaz, S., Paavonen, T., & Hayry, P. (1991). Chronic rejection in rat aortic allografts. An experimental model for transplant arteriosclerosis. *Arterioscler Thromb, 11*(3), 671-680.

Midwood, K., Sacre, S., Piccinini, A. M., Inglis, J., Trebaul, A., Chan, E., et al. (2009). Tenascin-C is an endogenous activator of Toll-like receptor 4 that is essential for maintaining inflammation in arthritic joint disease. *Nat Med, 15*(7), 774-780.

Midwood, K. S., & Orend, G. (2009). The role of tenascin-C in tissue injury and tumorigenesis. *J Cell Commun Signal, 3*(3-4), 287-310.

Mikalsen, B., Fosby, B., Wang, J., Hammarstrom, C., Bjaerke, H., Lundstrom, M., et al. (2010). Genome-wide transcription profile of endothelial cells after cardiac transplantation in the rat. *Am J Transplant, 10*(7), 1534-1544.

Mitchell, R. N. (2009). Graft vascular disease: immune response meets the vessel wall. *Annu Rev Pathol, 4*, 19-47.

Motamed, K., & Sage, E. H. (1998). SPARC inhibits endothelial cell adhesion but not proliferation through a tyrosine phosphorylation-dependent pathway. *J Cell Biochem, 70*(4), 543-552.

Murphy-Ullrich, J. E., Gurusiddappa, S., Frazier, W. A., & Hook, M. (1993). Heparin-binding peptides from thrombospondins 1 and 2 contain focal adhesion-labilizing activity. *J Biol Chem, 268*(35), 26784-26789.

Murphy-Ullrich, J. E., & Hook, M. (1989). Thrombospondin modulates focal adhesions in endothelial cells. *J Cell Biol, 109*(3), 1309-1319.

Murphy-Ullrich, J. E., Schultz-Cherry, S., & Hook, M. (1992). Transforming growth factor-beta complexes with thrombospondin. *Mol Biol Cell, 3*(2), 181-188.

Murphy, G. J., Bicknell, G. R., & Nicholson, M. L. (2003). Rapamycin inhibits vascular remodeling in an experimental model of allograft vasculopathy and attenuates associated changes in fibrosis-associated gene expression. *J Heart Lung Transplant, 22*(5), 533-541.

Nakahara, H., Gabazza, E. C., Fujimoto, H., Nishii, Y., D'Alessandro-Gabazza, C. N., Bruno, N. E., et al. (2006). Deficiency of tenascin C attenuates allergen-induced bronchial asthma in the mouse. *Eur J Immunol, 36*(12), 3334-3345.

Nishioka, T., Onishi, K., Shimojo, N., Nagano, Y., Matsusaka, H., Ikeuchi, M., et al. (2010). Tenascin-C may aggravate left ventricular remodeling and function after myocardial infarction in mice. *Am J Physiol Heart Circ Physiol, 298*(3), H1072-1078.

Nor, J. E., Mitra, R. S., Sutorik, M. M., Mooney, D. J., Castle, V. P., & Polverini, P. J. (2000). Thrombospondin-1 induces endothelial cell apoptosis and inhibits angiogenesis by activating the caspase death pathway. *J Vasc Res, 37*(3), 209-218.

Norris, R. A., Damon, B., Mironov, V., Kasyanov, V., Ramamurthi, A., Moreno-Rodriguez, R., et al. (2007). Periostin regulates collagen fibrillogenesis and the biomechanical properties of connective tissues. *J Cell Biochem, 101*(3), 695-711.

Norris, R. A., Moreno-Rodriguez, R., Hoffman, S., & Markwald, R. R. (2009). The many facets of the matricelluar protein periostin during cardiac development, remodeling, and pathophysiology. *J Cell Commun Signal, 3*(3-4), 275-286.

O'Regan, A. W., Chupp, G. L., Lowry, J. A., Goetschkes, M., Mulligan, N., & Berman, J. S. (1999). Osteopontin is associated with T cells in sarcoid granulomas and has T cell adhesive and cytokine-like properties in vitro. *J Immunol, 162*(2), 1024-1031.

Oka, T., Xu, J., Kaiser, R. A., Melendez, J., Hambleton, M., Sargent, M. A., et al. (2007). Genetic manipulation of periostin expression reveals a role in cardiac hypertrophy and ventricular remodeling. *Circ Res, 101*(3), 313-321.

Ono, K., & Lindsey, E. S. (1969). Improved technique of heart transplantation in rats. *J Thorac Cardiovasc Surg, 57*(2), 225-229.

Ophascharoensuk, V., Giachelli, C. M., Gordon, K., Hughes, J., Pichler, R., Brown, P., et al. (1999). Obstructive uropathy in the mouse: role of osteopontin in interstitial fibrosis and apoptosis. *Kidney Int, 56*(2), 571-580.

Patarca, R., Saavedra, R. A., & Cantor, H. (1993). Molecular and cellular basis of genetic resistance to bacterial infection: the role of the early T-lymphocyte activation-1/osteopontin gene. *Crit Rev Immunol, 13*(3-4), 225-246.

Poston, R. S., Billingham, M., Hoyt, E. G., Pollard, J., Shorthouse, R., Morris, R. E., et al. (1999). Rapamycin reverses chronic graft vascular disease in a novel cardiac allograft model. *Circulation, 100*(1), 67-74.

Prockop, D. J., & Kivirikko, K. I. (1995). Collagens: molecular biology, diseases, and potentials for therapy. *Annu Rev Biochem, 64*, 403-434.

Racanelli, A. L., Diemer, M. J., Dobies, A. C., Dubin, J. R., & Reilly, T. M. (1992). Comparison of recombinant plasminogen activator inhibitor-1 and epsilon amino caproic acid in a hemorrhagic rabbit model. *Thromb Haemost, 67*(6), 692-696.

Rentz, T. J., Poobalarahi, F., Bornstein, P., Sage, E. H., & Bradshaw, A. D. (2007). SPARC regulates processing of procollagen I and collagen fibrillogenesis in dermal fibroblasts. *J Biol Chem, 282*(30), 22062-22071.

Rhodes, J. M., & Simons, M. (2007). The extracellular matrix and blood vessel formation: not just a scaffold. *J Cell Mol Med, 11*(2), 176-205.

Rickenbacher, P. R., Kemna, M. S., Pinto, F. J., Hunt, S. A., Alderman, E. L., Schroeder, J. S., et al. (1996). Coronary artery intimal thickening in the transplanted heart. An in vivo intracoronary untrasound study of immunologic and metabolic risk factors. *Transplantation, 61*(1), 46-53.

Riser, B. L., Najmabadi, F., Perbal, B., Peterson, D. R., Rambow, J. A., Riser, M. L., et al. (2009). CCN3 (NOV) is a negative regulator of CCN2 (CTGF) and a novel endogenous inhibitor of the fibrotic pathway in an in vitro model of renal disease. *Am J Pathol, 174*(5), 1725-1734.

Riser, B. L., Najmabadi, F., Perbal, B., Rambow, J. A., Riser, M. L., Sukowski, E., et al. (2010). CCN3/CCN2 regulation and the fibrosis of diabetic renal disease. *J Cell Commun Signal, 4*(1), 39-50.

Rosenblatt, S., Bassuk, J. A., Alpers, C. E., Sage, E. H., Timpl, R., & Preissner, K. T. (1997). Differential modulation of cell adhesion by interaction between adhesive and counter-adhesive proteins: characterization of the binding of vitronectin to osteonectin (BM40, SPARC). *Biochem J, 324 (Pt 1)*, 311-319.

Ruegg, C. R., Chiquet-Ehrismann, R., & Alkan, S. S. (1989). Tenascin, an extracellular matrix protein, exerts immunomodulatory activities. *Proc Natl Acad Sci U S A, 86*(19), 7437-7441.

Sage, H., Vernon, R. B., Decker, J., Funk, S., & Iruela-Arispe, M. L. (1989). Distribution of the calcium-binding protein SPARC in tissues of embryonic and adult mice. *J Histochem Cytochem, 37*(6), 819-829.

Sato, I., & Shimada, K. (2001). Quantitative analysis of tenascin in chordae tendineae of human left ventricular papillary muscle with aging. *Ann Anat, 183*(5), 443-448.

Sawada, Y., Onoda, K., Imanaka-Yoshida, K., Maruyama, J., Yamamoto, K., Yoshida, T., et al. (2007). Tenascin-C synthesized in both donor grafts and recipients accelerates artery graft stenosis. *Cardiovasc Res, 74*(3), 366-376.

Scatena, M., Liaw, L., & Giachelli, C. M. (2007). Osteopontin: a multifunctional molecule regulating chronic inflammation and vascular disease. *Arterioscler Thromb Vasc Biol, 27*(11), 2302-2309.

Schellings, M. W., Pinto, Y. M., & Heymans, S. (2004). Matricellular proteins in the heart: possible role during stress and remodeling. *Cardiovasc Res, 64*(1), 24-31.

Schellings, M. W., Vanhoutte, D., Swinnen, M., Cleutjens, J. P., Debets, J., van Leeuwen, R. E., et al. (2009). Absence of SPARC results in increased cardiac rupture and dysfunction after acute myocardial infarction. *J Exp Med, 206*(1), 113-123.

Schiemann, B. J., Neil, J. R., & Schiemann, W. P. (2003). SPARC inhibits epithelial cell proliferation in part through stimulation of the transforming growth factor-beta-signaling system. *Mol Biol Cell, 14*(10), 3977-3988.

Schroen, B., Heymans, S., Sharma, U., Blankesteijn, W. M., Pokharel, S., Cleutjens, J. P., et al. (2004). Thrombospondin-2 is essential for myocardial matrix integrity: increased expression identifies failure-prone cardiac hypertrophy. *Circ Res, 95*(5), 515-522.

Schultz, G. S., & Wysocki, A. (2009). Interactions between extracellular matrix and growth factors in wound healing. *Wound Repair Regen, 17*(2), 153-162.

Serini, G., Bochaton-Piallat, M. L., Ropraz, P., Geinoz, A., Borsi, L., Zardi, L., et al. (1998). The fibronectin domain ED-A is crucial for myofibroblastic phenotype induction by transforming growth factor-beta1. *J Cell Biol, 142*(3), 873-881.

Shan, J., Huang, Y., Feng, L., Luo, L., Li, C., Ke, N., et al. (2010). A modified technique for heterotopic heart transplantation in rats. *J Surg Res, 164*(1), 155-161.

Shimazaki, M., Nakamura, K., Kii, I., Kashima, T., Amizuka, N., Li, M., et al. (2008). Periostin is essential for cardiac healing after acute myocardial infarction. *J Exp Med, 205*(2), 295-303.

Shinohara, M. L., Jansson, M., Hwang, E. S., Werneck, M. B., Glimcher, L. H., & Cantor, H. (2005). T-bet-dependent expression of osteopontin contributes to T cell polarization. *Proc Natl Acad Sci U S A, 102*(47), 17101-17106.

Sidhu, S. S., Yuan, S., Innes, A. L., Kerr, S., Woodruff, P. G., Hou, L., et al. (2010). Roles of epithelial cell-derived periostin in TGF-beta activation, collagen production, and collagen gel elasticity in asthma. *Proc Natl Acad Sci U S A, 107*(32), 14170-14175.

Strandjord, T. P., Madtes, D. K., Weiss, D. J., & Sage, E. H. (1999). Collagen accumulation is decreased in SPARC-null mice with bleomycin-induced pulmonary fibrosis. *Am J Physiol, 277*(3 Pt 1), L628-635.

Sun, Y., & Weber, K. T. (2005). Animal models of cardiac fibrosis. *Methods Mol Med, 117*, 273-290.

Takayama, G., Arima, K., Kanaji, T., Toda, S., Tanaka, H., Shoji, S., et al. (2006). Periostin: a novel component of subepithelial fibrosis of bronchial asthma downstream of IL-4 and IL-13 signals. *J Allergy Clin Immunol, 118*(1), 98-104.

Tamaoki, M., Imanaka-Yoshida, K., Yokoyama, K., Nishioka, T., Inada, H., Hiroe, M., et al. (2005). Tenascin-C regulates recruitment of myofibroblasts during tissue repair after myocardial injury. *Am J Pathol, 167*(1), 71-80.

Tamura, A., Shingai, M., Aso, N., Hazuku, T., & Nasu, M. (2003). Osteopontin is released from the heart into the coronary circulation in patients with a previous anterior wall myocardial infarction. *Circ J, 67*(9), 742-744.

Trueblood, N. A., Xie, Z., Communal, C., Sam, F., Ngoy, S., Liaw, L., et al. (2001). Exaggerated left ventricular dilation and reduced collagen deposition after myocardial infarction in mice lacking osteopontin. *Circ Res, 88*(10), 1080-1087.

Uzel, M. I., Scott, I. C., Babakhanlou-Chase, H., Palamakumbura, A. H., Pappano, W. N., Hong, H. H., et al. (2001). Multiple bone morphogenetic protein 1-related mammalian metalloproteinases process pro-lysyl oxidase at the correct physiological site and control lysyl oxidase activation in mouse embryo fibroblast cultures. *J Biol Chem, 276*(25), 22537-22543.

Waller, A. H., Sanchez-Ross, M., Kaluski, E., & Klapholz, M. (2010). Osteopontin in cardiovascular disease: a potential therapeutic target. *Cardiol Rev, 18*(3), 125-131.

Wang, J. C., Lai, S., Guo, X., Zhang, X., de Crombrugghe, B., Sonnylal, S., et al. (2010). Attenuation of fibrosis in vitro and in vivo with SPARC siRNA. *Arthritis Res Ther, 12*(2), R60.

Weber, G. F., Zawaideh, S., Hikita, S., Kumar, V. A., Cantor, H., & Ashkar, S. (2002). Phosphorylation-dependent interaction of osteopontin with its receptors regulates macrophage migration and activation. *J Leukoc Biol, 72*(4), 752-761.

Weiss, J. M., Renkl, A. C., Maier, C. S., Kimmig, M., Liaw, L., Ahrens, T., et al. (2001). Osteopontin is involved in the initiation of cutaneous contact hypersensitivity by inducing Langerhans and dendritic cell migration to lymph nodes. *J Exp Med, 194*(9), 1219-1229.

Winters, G. L. & Schoen, F. J. (2001). Pathology of cardiac transplantation. In M. D. Silver, G. A. I. & F. J. Schoen (Eds.), *Cardiovascular Pathology* (pp. 725-762): Churchill Livingstone.

Wipff, P. J., & Hinz, B. (2009). Myofibroblasts work best under stress. *J Bodyw Mov Ther, 13*(2), 121-127.

Wynn, T. A. (2008). Cellular and molecular mechanisms of fibrosis. *J Pathol, 214*(2), 199-210.

Xie, X. S., Li, F. Y., Liu, H. C., Deng, Y., Li, Z., & Fan, J. M. (2010). LSKL, a peptide antagonist of thrombospondin-1, attenuates renal interstitial fibrosis in rats with unilateral ureteral obstruction. *Arch Pharm Res, 33*(2), 275-284.

Yumoto, K., Ishijima, M., Rittling, S. R., Tsuji, K., Tsuchiya, Y., Kon, S., et al. (2002). Osteopontin deficiency protects joints against destruction in anti-type II collagen antibody-induced arthritis in mice. *Proc Natl Acad Sci U S A, 99*(7), 4556-4561.

Zhao, X. M., Hu, Y., Miller, G. G., Mitchell, R. N., & Libby, P. (2001). Association of thrombospondin-1 and cardiac allograft vasculopathy in human cardiac allografts. *Circulation, 103*(4), 525-531.

Zhou, Y., Poczatek, M. H., Berecek, K. H., & Murphy-Ullrich, J. E. (2006). Thrombospondin 1 mediates angiotensin II induction of TGF-beta activation by cardiac and renal cells under both high and low glucose conditions. *Biochem Biophys Res Commun, 339*(2), 633-641.

Part 3

Experimentation in Cardiac Transplantation

7

Potential of Heterotopic Cardiac Transplantation in Mice as a Model for Elucidating Mechanisms of Graft Rejection

Melanie Laschinger, Volker Assfalg, Edouard Matevossian, Helmut Friess and Norbert Hüser
Department of Surgery, Klinikum rechts der Isar, Technische Universität München, Germany

1. Introduction

Cardiac transplantation displays a well established therapeutic procedure for different end-stage heart diseases. Effective immunosuppressive drugs, progress in operative techniques, modern perioperative intensive care, and application of increasingly potent antibiotics in case of postoperative infections led to an improvement in short term outcome of organ transplantation. Nevertheless, achievements in long term transplant results are rare due to rejection of allografts. Chronic graft rejection is the major cause of late transplant failure.

According to present knowledge, T cells, infiltrating monocytes and macrophages, and NK cells, respectively, are involved in acute and chronic rejection. Numerous clinical trials and investigations in animal or cell culture models point out, that cell adhesion molecules, cytokines, and chemokines play a decisive role in the acute and chronic rejection of solid organ grafts.

Heterotopic cardiac transplantation in mice is considered to be the best model to study immunological mechanisms of transplant rejection. This technique allows the analysis of rejection processes in different mouse strains with defined genetic defects. Thus, distinct immunological receptors and ligands can be scrutinized for their impact on physiological and pathophysiological mechanisms of acute and chronic graft rejection. Results achieved from this model could be transferred to human beings in the majority of cases. As such, the model of heterotopic cardiac transplantation in mice has the potential to discover new therapeutic strategies which can be transferred to the clinic.

The aim of this chapter is to present our comprehensive microsurgical expertise on this model to other research groups in the field of cardiac transplantation. It delineates the practicable microsurgical model of heterotopic cardiac transplantation in mice as performed in our centre, based on the initially presented technique nearly four decades ago. Furthermore, the necessity of this *in vivo* model for a detailed understanding of the underlying mechanisms of transplant rejection is going to be discussed.

2. History and clinical-experimental development of transplantation

Basic requirement for transplantation of vascularized organs was the development of surgical vascular anastomosis techniques, crucially brought forward by Alexis Carrel in Lyon, France at the beginning of the last century [Carrel & Guthrie, 1905]. He successfully performed numerous heart transplantations in dogs and received the Nobel Prize for his research in 1912. In the year 1954 Joseph Murray (Boston, USA) performed the first successful solid organ transplantation in human beings in terms of the first kidney transplantation between monocygotic twins [Merrill et al., 1956]. In 1963 both Starzl (Denver, USA) and Hardy (Mississippi, USA) performed the first liver transplantation and lung transplantation, respectively. The first pancreas transplantation was realized by Richard Lillehei (Minnesota, USA) in 1966 and finally Christian Barnard (Cape Town, South Africa) performed the first human heart transplantation in 1967.

The knowledge about transplant immunology is derived from basic experimental findings during transplantation in animal models. Cellular principles of organ rejection were conclusively described by the English biologist Peter Medawar, who received the Nobel Prize for the "discovery of immunological tolerance" in 1960 [Billingham et al., 1951]. In 1953, histocompatibility antigen was reported for the first time on the surface of leucocytes. Jean Dausset therewith established the basis for histological typing between donor and recipient which is nowadays routinely performed within the pre-operative screening previous to each transplantation, the so-called HLA matching (testing of congruousness of those genes that are responsible for transplant rejection). Nevertheless, T cell mediated immune defence against the graft is not covered in these investigations though T cells take up a key function in transplant rejection [Sayegh & Carpenter, 2004]. This T cell reactivity could be accurately examined in our transplant centre in living donor kidney transplantation between monocygotic twins and in consequence immunosuppression was first reduced and then completely withdrawn [Hüser et al., 2009]. To date, medication free development of tolerance or at least reduction of required immunosuppressive drugs remains to be the unchanged goal for increased postoperative transplant survival.

Of course, transplantation of organs between genetically identical individuals continues to be exceptional as transplantation is usually performed in an allogeneic context which implicates the risk of an acute rejection episode. Technical advance and improvements in medicamentous therapy by implementation of potent immunosuppressants lead to an over-all one-year graft survival of more than 80% [Christie et al., 2010]. On the other hand, no relevant enhancements in long-term outcome of grafts could be determined. Chronic transplant rejection is hereby the main reason for late graft failure. Besides non-immunological donor- and recipient-dependent factors, mainly immunological reactions represent an important role for graft survival. Heterotopic heart transplantation in mice provides an important and valid model for analysis of immunological events during acute and chronic rejection mechanisms.

3. Necessity of an *in vivo* model for investigation of immunological events mediating organ rejection

The reaction against an allograft is composed of a complex cascade of immunological processes and some parts of them can be analyzed *in vitro*. However, detailed investigation of rejection mechanisms of vascularized grafts includes afferent and efferent steps like e.g. sensitisation of the recipient, antigen processing in lymphoid organs, differentiation and proliferation of immunocompetent cells of the recipient that detect the graft to be "extraneous" and finally direct their movement into the graft. These processes all culminate in graft failure, but they are not reproducible *in vitro*, because conclusion on the exact genesis and therefore identification of the causality of specific interactions is not possible. Experimental *in vivo* investigations are especially necessary to display the dynamic of these processes. The animal model is therefore an ideal compromise between clinical reality and experimental reproducibility. The study of genetically modified rodents has become commonplace within immunological research. Sophisticated advances in gene-altered models make it possible to appoint the function of a certain interaction of specific gene products in the context of graft rejection. Within these gene replacement (knock-in) or loss of function mutation (knock-out), mice have been generally accepted for both technical and nontechnical reasons. An observed phenotype can provide clues to the mechanisms of transplant immunology. Moreover, the use of inducible transgenic systems enables to control the location and time of transgene expression in certain tissues and avoids lethal deletion in knockout mice or compensation by various gene products. For evaluation of immunological and especially transplant immunological questions, results derived from the mouse model could directly be transferred to human beings for the most part, albeit the observations must be interpreted carefully due to some differences in both the innate and adaptive arm of the immune system [Mestas & Hughes, 2004]. A large number of important gene products that play an important role in this context were first defined in the mouse. Nearly all interaction molecules like T cell-receptors, cytokine-receptors, accessory molecules, and cell-activation-markers are characterized and a large number of genetically well-characterized transgenic and knock-out strains of the molecules are available. So far, use of homologous recombination to modify genes in embryonic stem cells was only feasible in mice because of the absenteeism of germline-competent embryonic stem cell lines in other species. Therefore, the murine model is more useful for the investigations of transplant rejection, although it requires a higher level of microsurgical skill than the technique in rats. It is only recently that Tong et al. have demonstrated stem cell based gene targeting technology in the rat [Tong et al., 2010]. Therefore the rat model might provide an adequate, powerful tool for the advancement of our understanding in transplant immunology in the future. The most frequently applied transplant model is still the heterotopic mouse heart transplantation. This procedure was described for the first time by Corry in 1973 [Corry et al., 1973] and the method was comparable to the cardiac transplantation in the rat as performed by Abbott et al. in 1964 [Abbott et al., 1964] and Ono et al. in 1969 [Ono & Lindsey, 1969].

A technique utilizing the transplantation of a non vascularized heart was established by Fulmer and coworkers, where neonatal murine cardiac tissue was placed subcutaneously into the pinna of the recipients ear [Fulmer et al., 1963]. Using this technique certain aspects of acute rejection have been studied. Nevertheless, the factors that lead to cardiac allograft vasculopathy all interact within the transplanted vessels at the blood / endothelial interface, making a vascularized cardiac transplant model imperative for the studies of chronic graft rejection [Hasagewa et al., 2007]. Other research groups refer to a simplified and technically easier model of vascularized transplantation in which the graft is anastomosed to the cervical vessels [Chen, 1991; Tomita et al., 1997]. However, according to Doenst et al., first, the positioning of the transplanted heart in an infrarenal position is self-guided and less likely to allow torsion, and second, the carotid artery is smaller in diameter than the ascending aorta of the donor, what makes the aorto-aortic anastomosis easier to perform [Doenst et al., 2001]. Finally the decision of which operative procedure is performed depends on the personal preference.

4. Anatomical specialities of the heterotopic heart transplantation model

The harvested donor heart is transplanted heterotopically by performing vascular anastomoses of the aorta and the pulmonary artery to the large infrarenal vessels of the recipient [Corry et al., 1973]. Therefore, the recipient mouse is not dependent on the functioning of the graft as its own heart remains untouched and the mouse undergoes rejection of the graft without impairment of physical well-being. A difference of this method compared to orthotopic heart transplantation is related to the technique of vessel anastomoses. The ascending aorta (AscA) of the donor heart is anastomosed end-to-side to the abdominal aorta (AbdA) and the pulmonary artery (PA) is anastomosed end-to-side to the recipient's inferior vena cava (IVC). This leads to a retrograde blood flow from the abdominal aorta via the ascending aorta directly into the coronary arteries whilst bypassing the left ventricle (LV) and left atrium (LA). After a while a thrombus accrues in the left ventricle. Hence, the oxygen supply of the heart muscle is hereby ensured by the capillary bed. Coming from the coronary arteries, the blood flow then passes the coronary veins and next converges in the coronary sinus (CS) and the right atrium (RA). From the right atrium the blood courses to the right ventricle (RV) and using the stump of the pulmonary trunk it finally reaches the recipients IVC (see *fig. 1*). The presented model is a so-called „non working heart model", because the graft does neither maintain physiological cardiac output nor pump against physiological pressure.

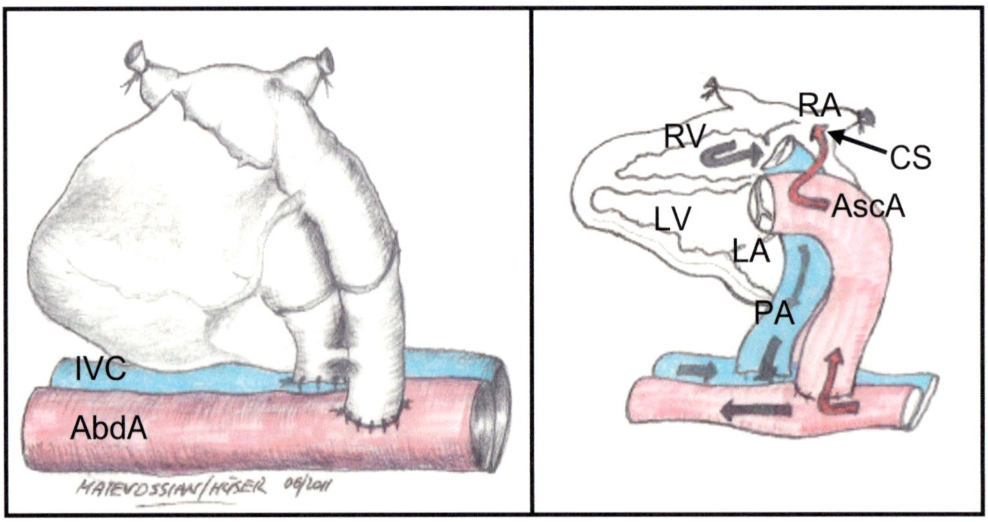

Fig. 1. Illustration of blood flow in heterotopically transplanted heart cardiac grafts

5. Options of rejection diagnostics after heterotopic heart transplantation

A relevant advantage of this operative method is the efficient rejection diagnostic of the transplanted heart. An algorithm on investigative technique could be developed to guarantee both the most comfortable examination for the transplanted mouse and the complete and comprehensive acquisition of acute and chronic rejection.

Finger palpation of the transplanted heart is a sensitive method to appraise time-dependent course of rejection. Concerning the contraction power and the induration of the graft, respectively, different stages can be graduated [Schmid et al., 1994]. In case of applying too high pressure, the graft cannot fill up and fully pulsate, and contractility is underestimated [Martins, 2008]. In the hand of an experienced diagnostician, slightest differences, especially the rapidly decreasing contraction power during acute rejection can be measured. In diagnostics of chronic transplant failure, evaluation occasionally might be difficult due to successive impairment of cardial pump functioning, as heart pulsation is directly related to the amount of intact myocard.

The validity of supplementary analysis to get the exact rejection time point remains controversial. Performance of electrocardiogram (ECG) requires exact subcutaneous placement of needle electrodes [Superina et al., 1986], validity is heavily dependent on the organ's position and movement [Mottram et al., 1988], and therefore the utility of this method is limited. In acute rejection, frequency shows rapid decrease in combination with various ECG alterations [Babuty et al., 1996]. In literature, magnetic resonance imaging is described as an additional tool in diagnostics for assessment of transplanted hearts. Nevertheless, this expensive procedure should be reserved for specific settings only. Moreover, in perfusion studies of solid grafts, results revealed to be extremely dependent on length and depth of narcosis [Wu et al., 2004]. Recent investigations describe high-frequency ultrasound biomicroscopy modality besides conventional echocardiography, a new non-invasive imaging method for diagnostic of acute rejection [Bishya, 2011]. Various papers report on a decrease of end-diastolic diameter and an increase of left ventricular posterior wall thickness, respectively, to be parameters of acute rejection. However, changes in left ventricular posterior wall thickness, seem to be increasingly difficult to measure after the fifth post-operative day, which points to the limitation of the use of echocardiogram in diagnosing acute allograft rejection [Scherrer-Crosbie et al., 2002]. In principle, every final rejection, either acute or chronic, has to be confirmed by diagnostic laparotomy to avoid misjudging passive movement of the graft by transmission of the aortic pulsation as graft beating.

6. The method of heterotopic heart transplantation in mice

The model of heterotopic heart transplantation in mice has been varied manifoldly since its first description by Robert Corry and Paul S. Russell in 1973 [Mao et al., 2009; Wang et al., 2005; Hasegawa et al., 2007]. The following chapter describes the transplantation procedure and incorporates our experience using an operating microscope (OPMI-6, Carl Zeiss, Jena, Germany) and a magnification between 4x-20x objective. Operation time is approximately 45 minutes and peri-operative mortality in the hands of an experienced micro-surgeon is less than 5%.

6.1 Anaesthesia and analgesia

All operative procedures in animals are performed using Isoflurane narcosis (Forene with 1-Chloro-2,2,2-trifluoroethyl-difluoromethylether). Both donor and recipient mouse can be operated under pain-free, unconscious, and relaxed conditions. Isoflurane narcosis brings along the crucial advantage of easy handling and having almost no influence on the animal's blood pressure in contrast to other narcotics such as e.g. Ketanest. Furthermore, Isoflurane narcosis is the least hepatotoxic narcotic drug. Basal anaesthesia is performed with 5% Isoflurane and for maintainance approximately 2% Isoflurane are necessary. Endotracheal anaesthesia is not necessary. Animals reliably wake up approximately 10 min after the end of narcosis.

6.2 Donor operation and preparation *ex situ*

The mouse intended for donor operation receives narcosis in the above mentioned way. Afterwards, the mouse which lies on its back gets fixed with tape at its limbs to a corkboard and Isoflurane is applied via a tube to the mouse's nose. Hereby, interim awakening of the animal can be avoided.

The operation starts with median laparotomy. The abdomen is kept open by use of two needles, fixing the peritoneum to the corkboard. The bowel gets enveloped into a moist compress and put away to the right side outside the mouse. Then the IVC and the abdominal aorta can be prepared with a cotton swab. Using 1 ml syringe and 25G needle, the Aorta is canulated and as much blood as possible is aspirated. The initially performed abdominal cut to the lower margin of the left hepatic lobe has to be extended to the sternum. Next, two more cuts have to be done along the costal arches to enable separation of the diaphragm from its costal and sternal adherence. In the following step the thorax is opened by cutting along the midaxillary line right up to the upper thorax aperture. Fixation of the sternum above the mouse's head (e.g. with a needle holder) guarantees free access to the opened thoracic cavity. Via puncture of the IVC the heart can now be flushed with cardioplegic fluid and it stops beating. After preparation and resection of the thymus gland, the inferior vena cava and the superior vena cava (SVC) are ligated with 6/0 silk. Silk ties are placed around the right and left pulmonary vessels (RPV / LPV) to exclude the lungs. Finally, the azygos vein (AV) is ligated. The donor heart is gently detached from the surrounding tissue with blunt dissection. For anastomosis of the recipient`s abdominal aorta (AbdA) the donor`s Aorta ascendens (AscA) and pulmonary artery (PA) remain open (see *fig.* 2). By now the heart can be harvested by sharply dividing along the esophagus and cutting the ligated vessels. The ascending aorta is cut below the brachiocephalic artery and the main pulmonary artery is cut proximal to its bifurcation.

Preparation of the pulmonary trunk and the Pars ascendens aortae has to be performed ex situ. Both of them are piggybacked on a curved pair of pincers and cut with a micro-surgical pair of scissors. Hereby you get two homogeneous and relatively long vessel stumps that enable easy implantation during the recipient operation. Until this moment the cardiac graft has to be stored in 4°C cold cardioplegic solution (e.g. Bretschneider's cardioplegic solution, Köhler Chemie, Alsbach, Germany).

6.3 Recipient preparation and transplantation

For the recipient operation narcosis, fixation on the corkboard, and median laparotomy from the symphysis to the lower margin of the left hepatic lobe are performed as described above during the donor operation. After opening the abdominal cavity and fixation of the peritoneum with two needles (alternatively a self-retaining retractor can be used) the bowel

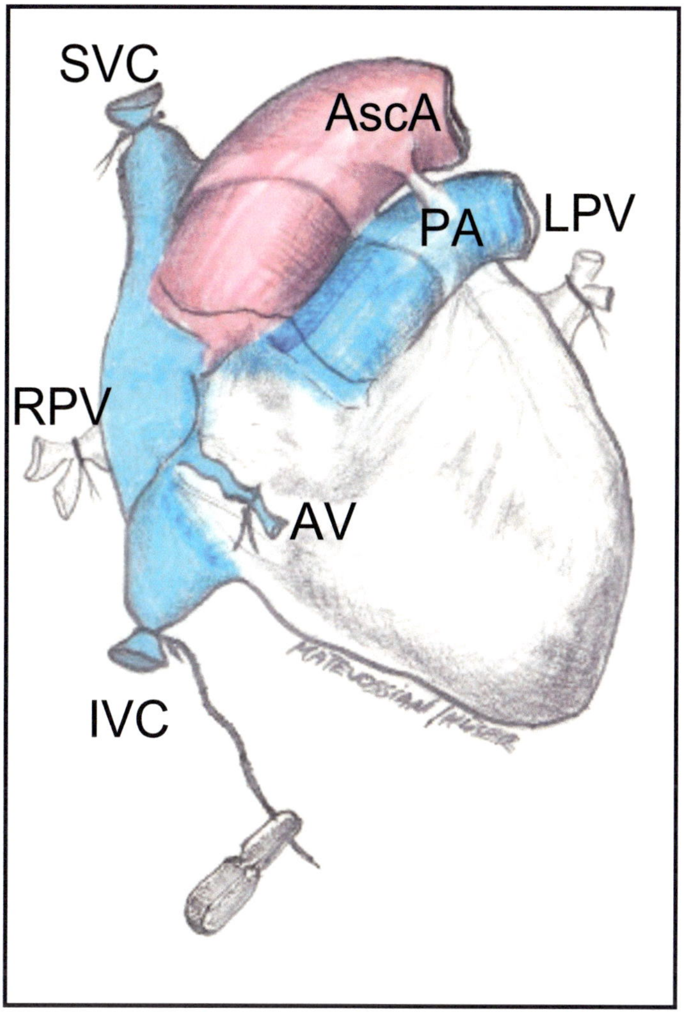

Fig. 2. Depiction of vascular ligatures at the donor's heart for organ harvesting

is enveloped into a moist compress and put away to the right side outside the mouse. Repetitive soaking of the compress with sterile saline guarantees a humid environment for the bowel during the entire procedure. The retroperitoneal space can be opened easily by gentle rotary motions with two cotton swabs. An additional cotton swab fixed in a needle holder can be used for permanent dislocation of the sigma and the left kidney outside the operating area after dividing the meso-sigmoid. Now the large vessels - Aorta abdominalis and IVC - are accessible and have to be separated from surrounding fatty tissue and adjacent lymph nodes. The preparation of the vessels starts directly below the outlet of the renal arteries and has to be performed to the aortic bifurcation. In case of lumbal veins in this segment, they have to be exposed and coagulated to assure that both the aorta and the IVC lie unfettered. Two vessel clamps have to be positioned at the ends of the prepared segment, respectively, to interrupt the flow in both the aorta and the IVC. The distal clamp has to be put first, to assure partially filled vessels for aortotomy and venotomy in the next step (see *fig.3*).

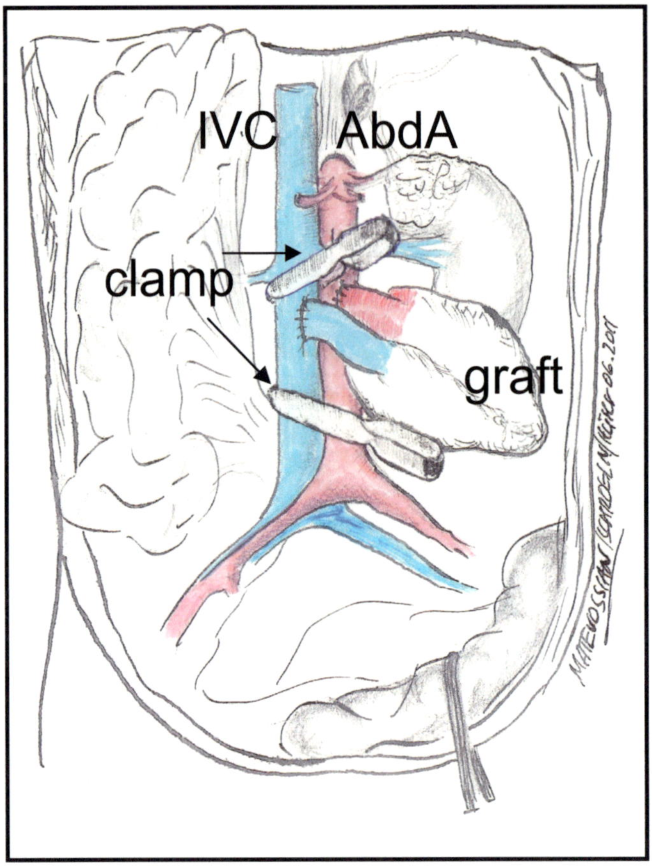

Fig. 3. Recipient preparation

After opening of the retroperitoneal space and positioning of the bowel which is enveloped into a moist compress and put away to the right side outside the mouse the colon sigmoideum and the left kidney are pulled away with a cotton swab fixed in a needle holder to guarantee free access to the Aorta abdominalis (AbdA) and the vena cava inferior (IVC). Two vascular clamps are positioned first just below the renal vessels and second at the proximal side of the bifurcation.

In the following step, the aorta has to be opened by a short longitudinal section using micro-scissors. This can be done easily without prior arteriotomy by a 25 or 30 gauge needle and is extended to a length of equal to the donor´s ascending aorta. After flushing the vascular lumen with saline, an end-to-side anastomosis of the pars ascendens aortae of the cardiac graft and the abdominal aorta has to be performed. The silk thread that has been left long at the IVC during the donor operation can now be inserted in a small clamp and therefore helps to move the heart without any injuring touch into the right position in relation to the recipient's vessels. Two stitches in the edges with a 10/0 monofil thread fix together the donor's and the recipient's aorta. The graft is shifted to the right inferior abdomen of the mouse to facilitate free access to the left lateral side of the aorta. Now the first continuous suture can be performed by means of 4 stitches. For the knot we use the thread of the opposite edge stitch (see *figure 4a*). At this time point the donor heart is flipped from the right side of the mouse to the left using the long thread at the IVC. The corkboard can now

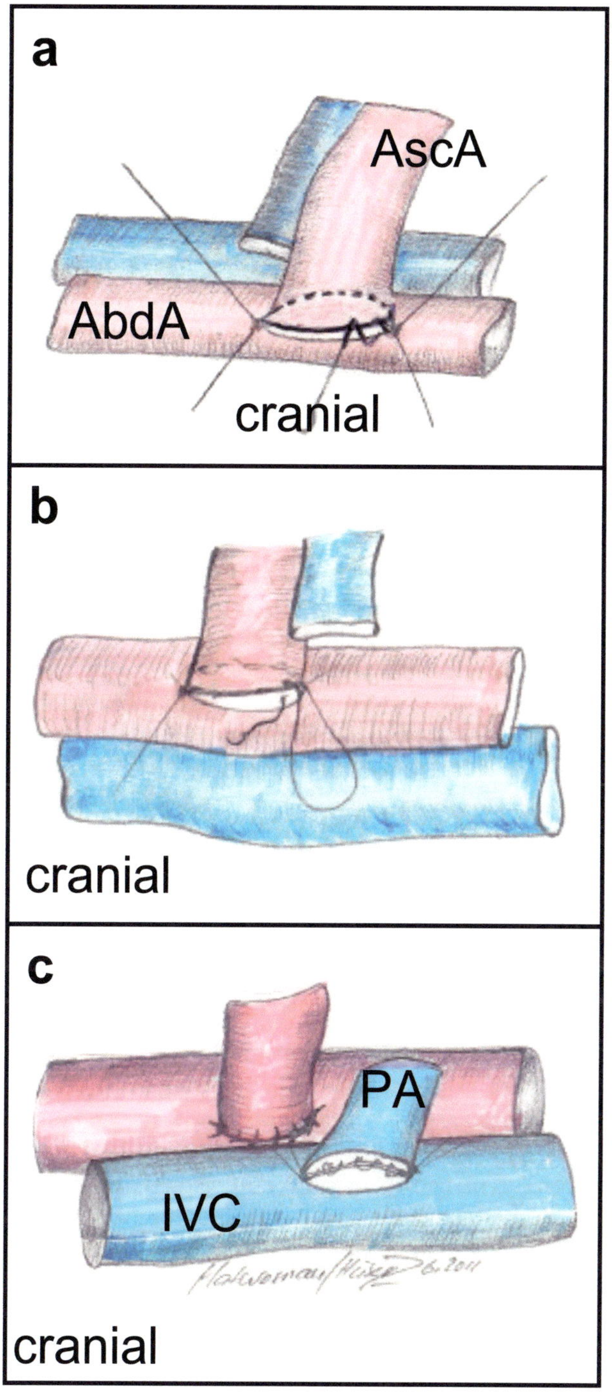

Fig. 4. Implantation of the vascularized graft
a) After flushing the vascular lumen with saline, the end-to-end anastomosis of the pars ascendens aortae of the cardiac graft (AscA) and the recipient's abdominal aorta (AbdA) is performed continuously with 4 stitches (direction of stitches: outside-inside / inside-

outside). Two edge stitches with a 10/0 monofile thread fix the donor's and the recipient's aorta. Gently tension to a thread of the ligature at the IVC of the graft enables easy positioning of the cardiac graft with regard to the recipients vessels.
b) The corkboard is turned and now the arterial "back-wall" becomes the "front-wall" which can be sutured continuously with 4 stitches (direction of stitches: outside-inside / inside-outside). The knot is done with the initially performed edge stitch and cut.
c) After venotomy again 2 edge stitches are necessary to adapt the pulmonary artery (PA) to the inferior vena cava (IVC). It is important to fix the "back wall" with slightly more tension compared to the "front wall" to obtain best possible exposition of the operation area. The first continuous suture is now performed inside the lumen (4 stitches, direction of stitches: inside-outside / outside-inside). Therefore the first stitch has to be performed from the outside to the inside and at the end of the suture the thread has to be stitched outside before knotting outside the vein's lumen. The last suture then can be performed continuously outside the vessel with 5 stitches at the "front wall" (direction of stitches: outside-inside / inside-outside).

be half-turned, so the vessel's "back wall" becomes "front wall" and the suture is performed accordingly with 4 stitches (see *figure 4b*). Finally, after knotting, the threads have to be cut to a length of approximately 2 mm. The next step is the venotomy. The incision with the micro scissors is performed just as the aortic incision and proportionately to the lumen of the pulmonary trunk of the donor. Again two edge stitches have to be done. Hereby it is important to fix the "back wall" with slightly more tension compared to the "front wall" to obtain best possible exposition of the operation area. This is due to the fact, that the end-to-side anastomosis of the opened IVC and the pulmonary artery of the donor has to be closed with a running suture in the inside of the IVC. For this purpose the suture must be stitched from the outside to the inside of the vessel lumen at the beginning and vice versa at the end of the suture before the knot can be done outside the lumen. For the continuous suture again 4 stitches are necessary (see *figure 4c*.)

After the knot with the proximal suture, the right wall of the IVC and the pulmonary artery of the donor are closed with another 5 stitches of a continuous suture outside the IVC. After knotting with the thread from the distal edge stitch both threads are cut to a length of approximately 2mm. Finally, the heart can be reperfused by opening the clamps after a cold ischemia period of approximately 25 minutes. The distal clamp is removed first to check the anastomosis of the IVC. Rapid stain towards bright red, refilling of the coronary vessels, and time-displaced beginning of cardiac contractions indicate the successful performance of the operation. After cleaning the heart from residual adjacent tissue particles and repositioning of the bowel into the abdominal cavity, the abdomen is closed by means of a continuous suture of the musculature and the peritoneum, respectively, and completing closure of the skin with single stitches (all using 5/0 monofil non-resorbable thread). Then the Isoflurane leading tube is removed from the animal's head. Within the next minutes the mouse awakes from narcosis. The recipient's operation takes approximately 35 minutes. The cage is put under a heating lamp for another 20 minutes and the recipient gets tramadol drops for post-operative analgesia.

7. Potential of heterotopic heart transplantation in mice for elucidating molecular mechanisms of graft rejection

Graduation of rejection after solid organ transplantation is primarily based on histopathological changes. Detection of immunological effector mechanisms display only a minor role in this field and cannot necessarily be correlated to the severity of graft rejection. Hyperacute, acute, and chronic rejections can be discriminated, but the impression must not be created that they are chronologically consecutive phases of rejection. Whereas hyperacute rejection emerges quite rapidly after transplantation, it is entirely possible, that acute and chronic rejection occur simultaneously. Therefore, each rejection episode is designated to a macroscopic and a histopathological image rather than to a concrete point in time (see also *fig.5*).

The molecular and cellular mechanisms of the innate and the adaptive immune system responsible for acute and chronic graft rejection have been studied in the experimental setting of heterotopic cardiac transplantation in detail. In vertebrates, innate immunity mediates early host defence and comprises inflammatory cells that express receptors detecting conserved pathogen associated molecular patterns (PAMPs). Beside non-cellular mediators capable of microbial recognition (e.g. the complement system) especially natural killer (NK) cells constantly participate in surveillance for intact self by sensing the presence of autologous major histocompatibility complex molecules. In this context we could demonstrate the importance of NK cells during rejection of cardiac transplants. Acute graft rejection includes massive NK and NKT cell infiltration into the transplanted organ. We found that NK and NKT cells, contribute to the activation of alloreactive T cells. Furthermore, inhibition of NK and/or NKT cells in absence of the co-stimulatory receptor CD28 induced long-term acceptance of semi-allogeneic grafts transplanted to CD28-deficient recipients [Maier et al., 2001]. In the same situation, fully allogeneic grafts were rejected in CD28 deficient hosts, although at later time point compared to wild type controls. These findings clearly point out the advantage of the *in vivo* model of cardiac transplantation allowing to create an either completely or semi-allogeneic constellation between donor and recipient. Importantly, the generation of allogeneic response against grafts involves numerous activation pathways and the impact of single components is often not visible unless this complexity is reduced. Moreover, NK1.1 positive (NK/NKT) cells could not only be assigned to have relevant influence on rejection of cardiac grafts, these data also hint to the important and close interaction between the innate and adaptive immune system.

The advances in immunosuppressive therapy have made severe acute cellular rejection of organ grafts uncommon. This has revealed to the form of acute antibody-mediated rejection – now widely accepted as a distinct clinicopathologic entity [Colvin, 2007] - that is resistant to current immunosuppression and acts through graft rejection by activation of complement, vascular endothelial and smooth muscle cells, and by activation of macrophages, neutrophils or NK cells, respectively [Wehner et al., 2009]. More recent data have highlightened antibody-mediated rejection as a cause for chronic rejection [Colvin, 2007]. A detailed knowledge of the underlying mechanism could provide insights for effective therapeutic interventions, e.g. monoclonal antibodies to C5 [Wang et al., 2007]. However, the use of the murine heart transplant model to determine whether antibodies contribute to the rejection process had only limited success so far [Wehner et al., 2009]. Anatomical differences of the cardiac vascular bed between humans and mice might be a limiting factor in addressing this particular question. In contrast to mice, human coronaries contain vasa vasorum, and coronaries of the murine heart do not pass the surface but rather directly enter the myocardium after their origin. Thus, investigating humoral rejection processes, the model of heterotopic heart transplantation in mice is only applicable to a limited range.

The adaptive immune response as an essential element of the rejection process is mainly characterized by an engagement of T cells. Genetically non-identical transplanted organs display peptides recognizes as foreign to host T cells. Helper T cells of the recipient become activated by foreign peptides that are displayed on antigen presenting cells (APC) in the donor organ. Interaction of activated helper T cells with B cells results in production of antibodies against the graft and activation of other immune cells, e.g. macrophages. In addition, allogen-specific CD8 cytotoxic T cells are known to be important for promoting transplant rejection in humans. This is in line with events during heterotopic allograft rejection in mice where we and others found a predominant activation of CD8 T cells in the transplanted heart of recipients [Hüser et al., 2010; Schnickel et al., 2004]. In vitro both, CD4 and CD8 T cells, proliferate in response to allogeneic stimuli. However, we could not detect activated CD4 T cells within cardiac grafts. In contrast, CD8 T cells were recruited in high numbers into the allograft and showed a phenotype of activated effector T cells [Hüser et al., 2010]. Again this indicates that the *in vivo* model of heterotopic heart transplantation in mice has great over *in vitro* studies and closely resembles the events taking place in humans.

Both, B and T lymphocytes use antigen receptor engagement to initiate distinct signal transduction pathways that affect cellular responses. It is well established that adaptor molecules regulate signaling of receptor proximal events inducing gene expression or cytoskeletal rearrangement. Beer et al. identified the putative adaptor protein SLY1, that is preferentially expressed in T and B lymphocytes and is defined as target for antigen receptor signal transduction with an important role in the adaptive immunity. It was shown that SLY mutant mice reveal impaired lymphoid organ development and antigen receptor mediated lymphocyte activation. Using the model of heterotopic cardiac transplantation, we were able to show extended allograft survival. Thus, signaling events mediated by SLY1 protein in cells of the adaptive immune system appear to be of importance for mechanisms inducing transplant rejection [Beer et al., 2005].

Chemokine receptors and their ligands, expressed by responding leukocytes and the inflamed transplant tissue, are responsible for the recruitment of alloreactive immunocytes into the graft. According to Hancock, several important points have emerged so far from murine *in vivo* transplant studies. (1) Targeting a single chemokine is in most cases ineffective in prolonging allograft survival, (2) chemokine receptors differ in their importance as targets in alloresponses, and (3) effects of concomitant immunosuppression can modulate the outcome of chemokine receptor targeting in otherwise untreated mice [Hancock, 2002]. The innate and adaptive immune reactions are initiated before, at the time of transplantation (e.g. by ischemia-reperfusion injury), and after transplantation by non-immunological and immunological factors, leading to graft vasculopathy with a diffuse narrowing of the coronary arteries and an adventitial fibrosis as common signs of chronic graft rejection. Chronic rejection is the response of the recipient's organism towards the cumulative injury to the transplanted graft over time, with involvement of cellular and humoral (antibody mediated) components [Chapman et al., 2005]. Best established model of chronic rejection in the mouse is the heterotopic cardiac allograft [Cornell et al., 2008]. On the basis of this *in vivo* model we could characterize the role of chemokine receptor CCR4 in chronic transplant failure. In accordance with Hancock [Hancock, 2002], absence of CCR4 receptor *per se* is not sufficient to achieve long-term transplant survival of fully allogeneic

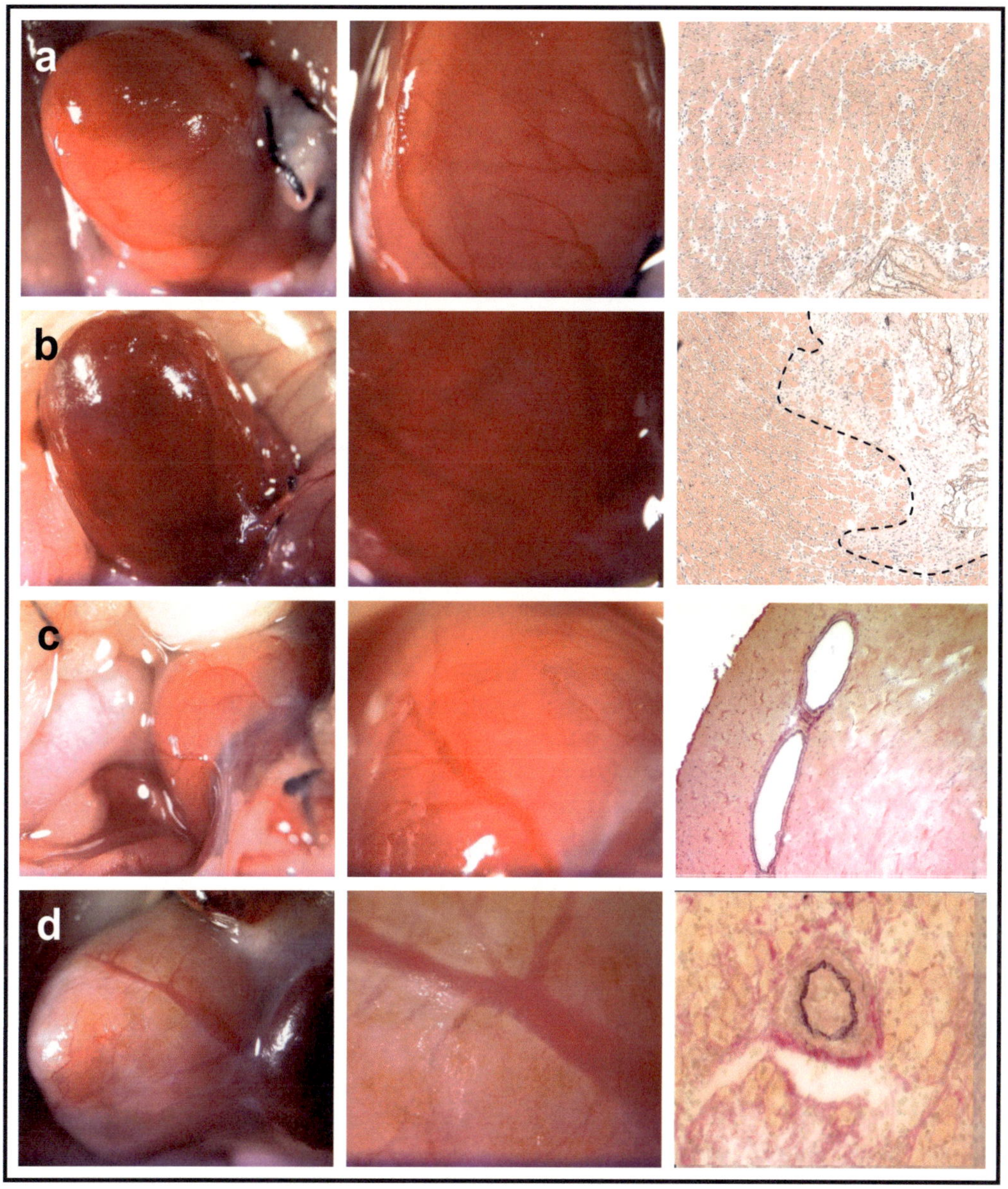

Fig. 5. Macro- and microscopy of transplanted hearts at different time points
a) syngeneic hearts 7 days post transplant and tissue section stained with haematoxylin and eosin, showing no signs of rejection, whereas in b) allografts 7 days post transplant display myocyte destruction by invading mononuclear cells, interstitial edema and necrosis (inflammatory lesion is highlighted within the dashed line), and macroscopically massive haemorrhage lesions, c) syngeneic grafts 100 days post transplant with slight adhesion to the surrounding tissue but microscopically normal vascular anatomy and d) chronic rejection in allografts with exhibition of transplant vasculopathy caused by excessive hyperplasia in the intima 100 days post transplant; a-b) HE staining at magnification x40, inflammatory lesion is highlighted in b, c-d) van Gieson staining at magnification x60.

donor hearts in CCR4-deficient recipients and only marginal prolongation of heart survival was noticed. In addition, no significant immunohistological difference in cellular infiltration comparing wild type and CCR4-deficient mice could be observed [Hüser et al., 2005]. In contrast, injection of Gallium nitrate, known to delay graft rejection, resulted in a significantly prolonged persistence of heart action in CCR4-deficient mice compared to wild type controls [Hüser et al., 2005]. These results could be confirmed by findings in CCL17-deficient mice, CCL17 being the specific ligand of CCR4 [Alferink et al., 2003]. Besides constitutively expressed chemokines like CCL19 and CCL21 that mainly recruit naive T cells in the lymph node, inflammatory chemokines like CCL2, CCL3, CCL17 and CCL22 mainly cause accumulation of activated T cells and T memory cells in inflamed organs. Inhibition of several of these chemokines have been shown to be beneficial for graft survival [Tan et al., 2005].

Recruitment of activated lymphocytes into inflamed tissue is of major importance for the control of immune responses. Beside chemokines, the role of the leukocyte integrins in the immunological reactions of organ transplant rejection is essential. The integrin LFA-1 is expressed on all leukocytes as an adhesion molecule and has a significant role not only in lymphocyte migration but also in mediating T cell interaction with APC and consequently T cell priming [Hogg et al., 2003]. Function of LFA-1 is tightly controlled by regulating its activity state [Evans et al., 2009]. Generating a mouse mutant that expresses constitutively active LFA-1 (LFA-$1^{d/d}$) [Semmrich et al., 2005] we could point out for the first time *in vivo* the importance of integrin deactivation on immune response inducing allograft rejection [IIüser et al, 2010]. We demonstrated that regulating LFA-1 activity from an active to an inactive state promotes successful activation, clonal expansion, and generation of effector T cells in response to allogeneic stimuli *in vivo*. Defective LFA-1 deactivation furthermore negatively affects recruitment of all major leukocytes from the innate and the adaptive immune system known to be involved in transplant rejection. By using the model of heterotopic cardiac transplantation we were able to provide direct *in vivo* evidence that regulating LFA-1 deactivation might be as important as regulating LFA-1 activation for effective immune responses during allograft rejection.

Those examples for studies in gene knock-out and transgenic mice using organ allografts identified the central role of a variety of target cells, chemotactic mediators, signalling components, and adhesion molecules on lymphocytes. As such, the described model of herterotopic cardiac transplantation in mice can be considered as a valid animal model and serves as an important achievement for clinical development of strategies that interfere with immune responses inducing transplant rejection.

8. Conclusion

Advances in the field of immunosuppression and better understanding of immunological courses in the last years contributed to establish organ transplantation as regularly performed clinical therapy and helped patients with severe renal, hepatic, pulmonary, and cardiac diseases to achieve longer survival and better quality of life. Short-term outcome after organ transplantation is impressive, whereas long-term graft survival remains to display a crucial problem. Induction of donor-specific tolerance towards transplanted tissue remains to bet the aim.

Heterotopic heart transplantation in mice is a vascularized immunological model and the recipient is not dependent on maintenance of circulation and cardiac functioning. As an *in vivo* model it has been shown to be an ideal compromise between clinical reality and experimental reproducibility of underlying essentials that peak in acute rejection or chronic transplant failure over time, however immunological differences between mice and human beings must be kept in mind. And, if so, mice as an *in vivo* model of first choice will continue to push forward our immunological understanding of immune reactions in transplantation.

9. References

Abbott, C.P., Lindsey, E.S., Creech, O. Jr. & Deitt, C.W. (1964). A technique for heart transplantation in the rat. *Arch Surg*, Vol. 89 (October 1964), 645-652.

Alferink, J., Lieberam. I., Reindl. W., Behrens. A., Weiss. S., Hüser, N., Gerauer, K., Ross, R., Reske-Kunz, A.B., Ahmad-Nejad, P., Wagner, H. & Förster, I. (2003). Compartmentalized production of CCL17 in vivo: strong inducibility in peripheral dendritic cells contrasts selective absence from the spleen. *J. Exp. Med*, Vol. 97, No. 5 (March 2003), 585–599.

Babuty, D., Aupart, M., Machet, M.C., Rouchet, S., Cosnay, P. & Garnier, D. (1996). Detection of acute cardiac allograft rejection with high resolution electrocardiography: experimental study in rats. *J Heart Lung Transplant*, Vol. 15, No. 11 (November 1996), 1120-1129.

Beer, S., Scheikl, T., Reis, B., Hüser, N., Pfeffer, K. & Holzmann, B. (2005). Impaired immune responses and prolonged allograft survival in Sly1 mutant mice. *Mol Cell Biol*, Vol. 25, No. 21 (November 2005), 9646-9660.

Billingham, R.E., Krohn, P.L. & Medawar, P.B. (1951). Effect of cortisone on survival of skin homografts in rabbits. *Br Med J*, Vol 2, No. 4739 (November 1951), 1157-1163.

Bishya, R.H. (2011). The "Mighty Mouse" Model in experimental cardiac transplantation. *Hypothesis*, Vol. 9, No 1, e5.

Carrel, A. & Guthrie, C.C. (1905). Functions of transplanted Kidney. *Science*, Vol. 22, No. 563, (October 1905), 473.

Chapman, J.R., O'Connell, P.J. & Nankivell, B.J. (2005). Chronic renal allograft dysfunction. *J Am Soc Nephrol*, Vol. 16, No. 10 (October 2005), 3015-3026.

Chen, Z.H. (1991). A technique of cervical heterotopic heart transplantation in mice. Transplantation, Vol. 52, No. 6 (December 1991), 1099-1101

Christie, J.D., Edwards, L.B., Kucheryavaya, A.Y., Aurora, P., Dobbels, F., Kirk, R., Rahmel, A.O., Stehlik, J. & Hertz, M.I. (2010). The Registry of the International Society for Heart and Lung Transplantation: twenty-seventh official adult lung and heart-lung transplant report--2010. *J Heart Lung Transplant*, Vol. 29, No. 10 (October 2010), 1104-1118.

Colvin, R.B. (2007). Antibody-mediated renal allograft rejection: diagnosis and pathogenesis. *J. Am. Soc. Nephrol*, Vol. 18, No. 4 (April 2007), 1046–1056.

Cornell, L.D., Smith, R.N. & Colvin, R.B. (2008). Kidney transplantation: mechanisms of rejection and acceptance. *Annu Rev Pathol*, Vol. 3, 189-220.

Corry, R.J., Winn, H.J. & Russell, P.S. (1973). Primarily vascularized allografts of hearts in mice. The role of H-2D, H-2K, and non-H-2 antigens in rejection. *Transplantation,* Vol. 16, No. 4 (October 1973), 343-350.

Doenst, T., Schlensack, C., Kobba J.L. & Beyersdorf, F. (2001). A technique of heterotopic, infrarenal heart transplantation with double anastomosis in mice. *J Heart Lung Transplant,* Vol. 20, No. 7 (July 2001), 762-765.

Dooms, H. & Abbas, A.K. (2006). Control of CD4+ T-cell memory by cytokines and costimulators. *Immunol. Rev,* Vol. 211 (June 2006), 23–38.

Evans, R., Patzak, I., Svensson, L., De Filippo, K., Jones, K., McDowall, A. & Hogg, N. (2009). Integrins in immunity. *J Cell Sci,* Vol. 122 (January 2009), 215-225.

Fulmer, R.I., Cramer, A.T., Liebelt, R.A. & Liebelt, A.G. (1963). Transplantation of cardiac tissue into the mouse ear. *Am J Anat,* Vol. 113 (September 1963), 273-285.

Hancock, W.W. (2002). Chemokines and transplant immunobiology. *J Am Soc Nephrol,* Vol. 13, No. 3 (March 2002), 821-824.

Hasegawa, T., Visovatti, S.H., Hyman, M.C., Hayasaki, T.& Pinsky, D.J. (2007). Heterotopic vascularized murine cardiac transplantation to study graft arteriopathy. *Nat Protoc,* Vol.2, No. 3, 471-480.

Hogg, N., Laschinger, M., Giles, K. & McDowall, A.(2003). T-cell integrins: more than just sticking points. *J Cell Sci,* Vol 116, No. 23 (December 2003), 4695-4705.

Hüser, N., Tertilt, C., Gerauer, K., Maier, S., Traeger, T., Assfalg, V., Reiter, R., Heidecke, C.D. & Pfeffer, K. (2005). CCR4-deficient mice show prolonged graft survival in a chronic cardiac transplant rejection model. *Eur J Immunol,* Vol. 35, No. 1 (January 2005), 128-138.

Hüser, N., Matevossian, E., Schmidbauer, P., Assfalg, V., Scherberich, J.E., Stangl, M., Holzmann, B., Friess, H. & Laschinger, M. (2009). Calculated withdrawal of low-dose immunosuppression based on a detailed immunological monitoring after kidney transplantation between monocygotic twins. *Transpl Immunol,* Vol. 22, No. 1-2 (December 2009), 38-43.

Hüser, N., Fasan, A., Semmrich, M., Schmidbauer, P., Holzmann, B & Laschinger, M. (2010). Intact LFA-1 deactivation promotes T-cell activation and rejection of cardiac allograft. *Int Immunol,* Vol. 22, No. 1 (January 2010), 35-44.

Maier, S., Tertilt, C., Chambron, N., Gerauer, K., Huser, N., Heidecke, C.D. & Pfeffer, K. (2001). Inhibition of natural killer cells results in acceptance of cardiac allografts inCD28−/− mice. *Nat. Med,* Vol 7, No. 5 (May 2001), 557–562.

Mao, M., Liu, X., Tian, J., Yan, S., Lu, X., Gueler, F., Haller, H. & Rong, S. (2009). A novel and knotless technique for heterotopic cardiac transplantation in mice. *J Heart Lung Transplant,* Vol. 28, No. 10 (October 2009), 1102-1106.

Martins, P.N. (2008). Assessment of graft function in rodent models of heart transplantation. *Microsurgery.,* Vol. 28, No. 7, 565-570.

Mestas, J. & Hughes, C.C. (2004). Of mice and not men: differences between mouse and human immunology. *J Immunol,* Vol. 172, No. 5 (March 2004), 2731-2738

Merrill, J.P., Murray, J.E., Harrison, J.H. & Guil, W.R. (1956). Successful homotransplantations of the human kidney between identical twins. *J Am Med Assoc,* Vol. 160, No. 4 (January 1956), 277-282.

Mottram, P.L., Smith, J.A., Mason, A., Mirisklavos, A., Dumble, L.J. & Clunie, G.J. (1988). Electrocardiographic monitoring of cardiac transplants in mice. *Cardiovasc Res*, Vol. 22, No. 5 (May 1988), 315-321.

Ono, K. & Lindsey, E.S. (1969). Improved technique of heart transplantation in rats. *J Thorac Cardiovasc Surg*, Vol 57, No. 2 (February 1969), 225-229.

Sayegh, M.H. & Carpenter, C.B. (2004). Transplantation 50 years later - progress, challenges, and promises. *N Engl J Med*, Vol. 351, No. 26 (December 2004), 2678-2680.

Scherrer-Crosbie, M., Glysing-Jensen, T., Fry, S.J., Vançon, A.C., Gadiraju, S., Picard, M.H. & Russell, M.E. (2002). Echocardiography improves detection of rejection after heterotopic mouse cardiac transplantation. *J Am Soc Echocardiogr*, Vol. 15, No. 10 (October 2002), 1315-1320.

Schmid, C., Binder, J., Heemann, U. & Tilney, N.L. (1994). Successful heterotopic heart transplantation in rat. *Microsurgery*, Vol. 15, No. 4, 279-281.

Schnickel, G.T., Whiting, D., Hsieh, G.R., Yun, J.J, Fischbein, M.P., Yao, W., Shfizadeh, A. & Ardehali, A. (2004). CD8 lymphocytes are sufficient for the development of chronic rejection. *Transplantation*, Vol. 78, No. 11 December 2004), 1634-1639.

Semmrich, M., Smith, A., Feterowski, C., Beer, S., Engelhardt, B., Busch, D.H., Bartsch, B., Laschinger, M., Hogg, N., Pfeffer, K. & Holzmann, B. (2005). Importance of integrin LFA-1 deactivation for the generation of immune responses. *J Exp Med*, Vol. 201, No. 12 (June 2005), 1987-1998.

Superina, R.A., Peugh, W.N., Wood, K.J. & Morris, P.J. (1986). Assessment of primarily vascularized cardiac allografts in mice. *Transplantation*, Vol. 42, No. 2 (August 1986), 226-227.

Tan, J., Zhou, G. (2005). Chemokine receptors and transplantation. *Cell Mol Immunol*, Vol. 2, No. 5 (October 2005), 343-349.

Tomita, Y., Zhang, Q.W., Yoshikawa, M., Uchida, T., Nomoto, K. & Yasui, H. (1997). Improvd technique of heterotopic
cervical heart transplantation in mice. *Transplantation*, Vol. 64, No. 11 (December 1997), 1598-1601.

Tong, C., Li, P., Wu, N.L., Yan, Y. and Ying, Q.L. (2010). Production of p53 gene knockout rats by homologous recombination in embryonic stem cells. *Nature*, Vol.9, No. 467 (September 2010), 211-213.

Wang, Q., Liu, Y., Li, X.K. (2005). Simplified technique for heterotopic vascularized cervical heart transplantation in mice. *Microsurgery*, Vol. 25, No. 1, 76-79.

Wang, H., Arp, J., Liu, W., Faas, S.J., Jiang, J., Gies, D.R., Ramcharran, S., Garcia, B., Zhong, R. & Rother, R.P. (2007). Inhibition of terminal complement components in presensitized transplant recipients prevents antibody-mediated rejection leading to long-term graft survival and accommodation. *J Immunol*, Vol. 179, No. 7 (October 2007), 4451–4463.

Wehner, J.R., Morrell, C.N., Rodriguez, E.R., Fairchild, R.L. & Baldwin, W.M. 3rd. (2009). Immunological challenges of cardiac transplantation: the need for better animal models to answer current clinical questions. *J Clin Immunol*, Vol. 29, No. 6 (November 2009), 722-729.

Wu, Y.J., Sato, K., Ye, Q. & Ho, C. (2004). MRI investigations of graft rejection following organ transplantation using rodent models. *Methods Enzymol*, Vol. 386, 73-105.

8

Pre-Transplant Therapy in Experimental Heart Transplantation

Tomislav Stojanovic[1], Andreas H. Wagner[2], Friedrich A. Schöndube[1] and Markus Hecker[2]
[1]*Department of Cardiovascular and Thoracic Surgery, University of Göttingen, Göttingen,*
[2]*Institute of Physiology and Pathophysiology, Division of Cardiovascular Physiology, University of Heidelberg, Heidelberg,*
Germany

1. Introduction

Heart transplantation is a life-saving procedure for patients with end-stage cardiac dysfunction. Currently one-year graft survival ranges between 77-88%, three-year survival between 77-79% and five-year survival between 67-73% (http://www.americanheart.org/presenter.jhtml?identifier=4588). Despite these encouraging results, primary graft failure accounts for about 23% of deaths in the first 90 days post transplantation. Pretransplant variables associated with primary graft failure include: ischemia time, donor gender, donor age, multiorgan donation, center volume, extracorporeal membrane oxygenation, mechanical circulatory support, etiology of heart failure, and reoperative heart transplantation (Russo et al., 2010). To target rejection of allografts, a variety of immunosuppressive protocols are used solely in the recipient who is the main focus of the therapy (The International Society of Heart and Lung Transplantation Guidelines for the Care of Heart Transplant Recipients Task Force 2: Immunosuppression and Rejection (Nov. 8, 2010)). Typically, neither donor nor grafts are specifically treated before or during organ harvesting except for the maintenance of circulatory and respiratory functions of the donor and irrigation of grafts with preservation solutions.

2. Graft rejection

A T-cell driven process mediated by the adaptive immune system is our classic understanding of graft rejection. Allogeneic MHC molecules on graft tissue are recognized by the recipient's immune system by two pathways, the direct and the indirect pathway. Alloreactive T-cells in the direct pathway recognize donor MHC molecules on antigen-presenting cells (APCs) which pass through the transplanted tissues (Larsen et al., 1990). APCs in the indirect pathway process antigens which are derived from donor MHC molecules and present them to alloreactive T-cells (Game & Lechler, 2002). Their activation is further fuelled by co-stimulatory molecules such as the CD40-CD40 ligand (CD154) receptor-ligand pathway (Cho et al., 2000). This co-stimulation, in case of graft endothelial cells, not only reinforces T-cell activity but enhances the later recruitment of effector leukocytes, namely monocytes (Rose, 1997). Leukocyte-endothelial cell interaction, thus exaggerated, causes damage to the capillary microcirculation, organ dysfunction and ultimately graft loss (Cho et al., 2000; Rocha et al., 2003).

Although T-cells are believed to play a critical role in acute rejection, it could be shown that expression of pro-inflammatory mediators within the allograft is up-regulated even before the T-cell response. This response is mediated by the innate immune system which is independent of the adaptive immune reaction (Christopher et al., 2002; He et al., 2002; He et al., 2003). By means of RNase protection assay in a mouse heart transplantation model it has been shown that one day after transplantation the gene expression profile of the cellular infiltrate, namely chemokine receptor expression and the expression of pro-inflammatory cytokines, was similar in RAG-deficient mice as compared to immunologically competent wild type mice (He et al., 2002). It could therefore be concluded that innate, antigen-independent pro-inflammatory processes occur shortly after transplantation and are further specifically modified by the adaptive immune response (He et al., 2003).

3. Innate immune system and ischemia reperfusion in organ transplantation

Multicellular organisms have developed immunological mechanisms to detect and to rapidly respond to threats. Such immunological mechanisms are being referred to as innate immunity. Unlike the evolutionary younger adaptive immune system, the innate immune system performs its control function by using so-called "pattern recognition" receptors (PRRs) (Janeway & Medzhitov, 2002). PRRs identify pathogenic molecules, microbial "non-self" (pathogen-associated molecular patterns [PAMP]) or recipient molecules released from damaged or "stressed" tissues ("damaged self" or damage-associated molecular patterns [DAMP]) that differ from "self" which are thought to signal through PRRs such as toll-like receptor 4 (TLR4) in a manner similar to PAMPs (Mollen et al., 2006).

Different cell types play a role in the effector response, among others dendritic cells, natural killer cells and endothelial cells. They detect PAMPs as exogenous and DAMPs as endogenous ligands through toll-like receptors (Land, 2003; Land, 2005; Takeda & Akira, 2005) (Figure 1).

Engagement of DAMPs with TLRs leads to activation of transcription factors STAT-1, AP-1, NF-κB and IRF-3 followed by chemokine (e.g. MCP-1) and pro-inflammatory cytokine release, graft damage and ultimately graft loss.

After recognition of PAMPs the activated TLRs initiate an intracellular signalling cascade which leads to activation of transcription factors such as, e.g. activator protein-1 (AP-1), nuclear factor-κB (NF-κB) or interferon regulatory factor-3 (IRF-3), expression of pro-inflammatory genes and, e.g. maturation of dendritic cells (Ishitani et al., 2003; Hemmi & Akira, 2005; Kishida et al., 2005; Sato et al., 2005; Shim et al., 2005; Takeda & Akira, 2005). Mature dendritic cells interact with naïve T-cells and trigger a T-cell response. They act therefore as a link between innate and adaptive immunity.

The process of organ injury starts even before the recipient's immune system has the first contact with donor cells. Its starts with the oxidative damage to the graft in the brain-dead donor and continues after reperfusion (Land, 2005). NADPH oxidase-dependent reactive oxygen species (ROS) production is involved in translocation of TLR4 to lipid rafts (Nakahira et al., 2006), i.e. micro-domains of the cell membrane, a process that is important

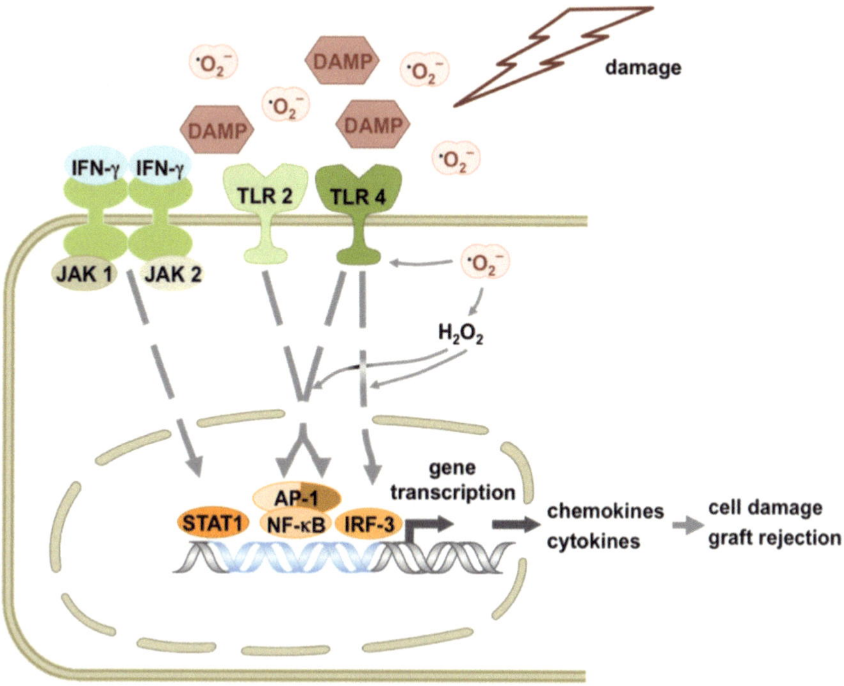

Fig. 1. Scheme of the innate immunity effector response after challenge by DAMPs (modified after Land 2007 (Land, 2007)).

in signal transduction (Dykstra et al., 2003; Manes et al., 2003). DAMPs like heat shock protein 72 (HSP 72), high mobility group box 1 (HMGB-1) and fragments of hyaluronic acid (fHA) are recognised by TLR4 and/or TLR2 (Land, 2007). Activation of these TLRs initiates a signal transduction cascade to the nucleus through molecules like myeloid differentiation marker 88 (MyD88), TIR-associated protein (TIRAP) und TIR domain-containing adaptor inducing IFN-β (TRIF), ultimately leading to activation of the transcription factors AP-1, NF-kB or IRF-3, up-regulation of pro-inflammatory gene expression and, among others, maturation of dendritic cells that all fuel the immunologic reaction against the graft (Land, 2007).

In summary, ROS in the brain-dead donor and during reperfusion cause i) initial graft damage which activates the innate immune response, ii) activation of signalling pathways which further augment this response and iii) boosting of humoral, complement-mediated tissue damage (Land, 2007).

4. Graft rejection and endothelial cells

In the setting of graft rejection, endothelial cells are the first donor cells which are affected by activation of the innate and adaptive immune response of the recipient. Integrity of the donor endothelium is of pivotal importance to graft function because injury to the endothelium ultimately leads to perfusion failure and graft loss. In addition, the endothelial cells themselves activate the innate immune response thereby maintaining a vicious circle (Rose, 1997; Rose, 1998; Methe et al., 2007). Graft injury due to ROS and activation of the innate immune response occurs very early at the level of the donor endothelial cells. In this context, systemic immunosuppressive therapy has the disadvantage of being initiated in the recipient while graft damage is already in transition and furthermore it does not specifically target endothelial cell damage. In fact, it may even augment it. Therefore, an adjunct pre-transplant therapy solely within the graft that addresses the pro-inflammatory effects of the innate immune response on the endothelium seems to hold great promise. Moreover, by excluding systemic effects, the therapy can be adequately dosed and administered directly to the target site because the graft vessels are readily accessible after organ explantation.

5. Decoy oligodeoxynucleotide technology in organ transplantation

To specifically address this setting, the decoy oligodeoxynucleotide (ODN) technology may provide a specific tool to directly interfere with target gene expression. Decoy (decoy=bait) ODNs are short double-stranded DNA molecules with a specific sequence of bases that typically matches the consensus DNA recognition motif of the target transcription factor. With these nucleic acid-based drugs it is possible to effectively inhibit the expression of genes which are controlled by the said transcription factor (Morishita et al., 1995). Most mammalian cells are easily transfected with these DNA molecules. In fact, their uptake by most target cells does not require any transfection agent or the like, and under physiological conditions is mediated by active transport, i.e. a carrier system and/or receptor mediated endocytosis (Figure 2).

The synthetic, 15 to 25 bp long DNA fragments usually are stabilized by replacing 2 to 3 of the terminal phosphodiester bonds between the nucleotides by phosphothio-ester bonds

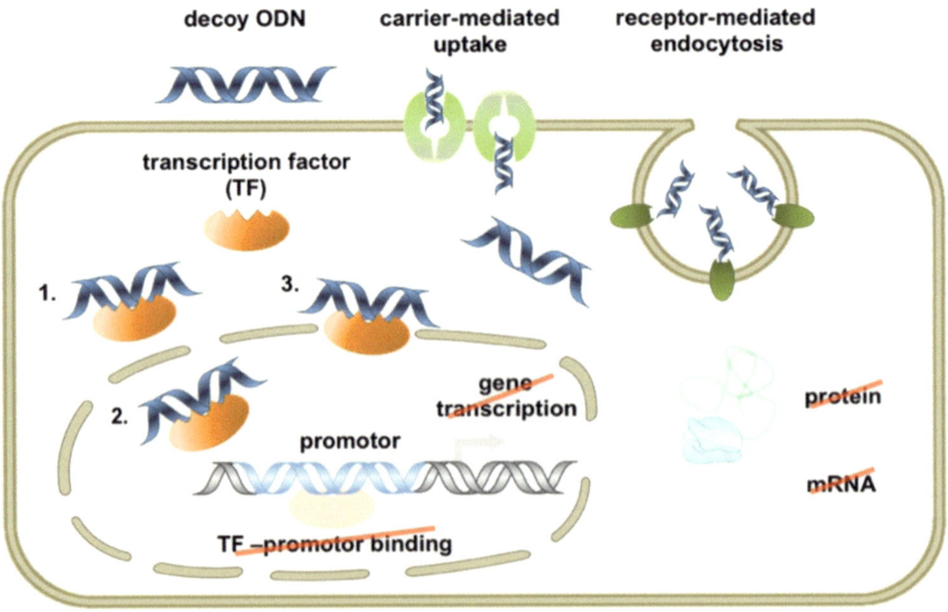

Fig. 2. Decoy ODN mechanism of action. Scheme depicting the mechanism of action of decoy ODN-mediated neutralization of the targeted transcription factor (TF). 1 refers to cytoplasmic TF sequestration, 2 to nuclear TF sequestration, and 3 to removal of promotor-bound TF through titration with high-affinity decoy ODNs.

that afford remarkable protection against exonucleases so that they remain intact in the target cells for some days. As mentioned above, decoy ODNs typically harbour at least one binding site for a particular transcription factor or transcription factor family. The length of this binding site normally is derived from known DNA binding motifs for the target transcription factor in different species and on the basis of their homology (consensus sequence).

Following their uptake by the respective target cell(s), decoy ODNs bind to their target transcription factor with high affinity (comparable to the formation of an antigen-antibody complex) thereby preventing it from translocation to the nucleus and/or effectively neutralizing its activity therein.

6. Role of interferon-γ and signal transducer and activator of transcription-1 (STAT-1) in transplant rejection

Acute cellular rejection reduces the short and long-term outcome after transplantation. Recipient immune cells are recruited from the circulation into the transplant by presentation of antigens to T-helper cells whose activation is further increased by co-stimulatory molecules such as the CD40-CD154 receptor-ligand pathway (Cho et al., 2000). As a consequence, activated T-helper cells induce the increased expression of adhesion molecules on the endothelial cells of the donor organ, which leads to further recruitment of circulating monocytes into the graft and ultimately graft failure (Cho et al., 2000).

An important cytokine that is produced by activated T-helper cells is interferon-γ (IFN-γ). Due to activation of the transcription factor signal transducer and activator of transcription-1 (STAT-1) IFN-γ up-regulates the expression of a number of important genes for graft rejection in the endothelial cells of the donor organ such as, e.g. vascular cell adhesion molecule-1 (VCAM-1) or CD40 (De Caterina et al., 2001; Wagner et al., 2002). VCAM-1 expression, for example, fuels leukocyte-endothelial cell interaction which is a hallmark of acute vascular rejection (De Caterina et al., 2001; Wagner et al., 2002).

Signalling of IFN-γ to the nucleus of an endothelial cell starts with its binding to the corresponding receptor on the cell surface which then dimerizes (Bach et al., 1997; Boehm et al., 1997; Pestka, 1997). As a consequence, the receptor-associated tyrosine kinases JAK1 and JAK2, members of the Janus family of kinases (Boehm et al., 1997; Pestka, 1997), translocate to the cell membrane. There they phosphorylate the cytoplasmic domain of the IFN-γ receptor which is now able to recruit monomeric STAT-1 (Ivashkiv, 1995; Ihle, 1996; Darnell, 1997). After phosphorylation and dimerization the now active transcription factor translocates to the nucleus and stimulates IFN-γ-dependent gene expression by binding to the gamma-interferon-activated element (GAS) in the promoter region of its target genes (Ivashkiv, 1995; Ihle, 1996; Darnell, 1997). In addition to CD40, the expression of ICAM-1 (Naik et al., 1997) or that of the inducible isoform of nitric oxide (NO) synthase is also controlled by STAT-1 (Ganster et al., 2001).

IFN-γ as a multifunctional cytokine therefore controls many pro-inflammatory gene products whose expression is stimulated through the IFN-γ/STAT-1 pathway (Khabar et al., 2004; Khabar & Young, 2007; Liu et al., 2008; Karonitsch et al., 2009). *In vivo* and *in vitro* experiments showed that the up-regulation of both CD40 and VCAM-1 expression by STAT-1 is effectively reduced using decoy ODNs directed against this transcription factor (Wagner et al., 2002; Quarcoo et al., 2004).

The role of CD40-CD154 co-stimulation in transplant rejection still is the subject of intense research (Larsen & Pearson, 1997; Cho et al., 2000). Thus it was shown in human biopsies of heart transplants that there is a significant correlation between the increased expression of CD154 and CD40 on leukocytes and endothelial cells, respectively, and acute rejection (Reul et al., 1997). The administration of monoclonal antibodies directed against CD154 prolonged renal transplant survival in rats and primates (Gudmundsdottir & Turka, 1999; Hancock, 1999; Kirk et al., 1999). Furthermore, the application of anti-CD40 antibodies in monkeys led to a significant immunosuppressive effect and prolonged graft survival (Imai et al., 2007), so that both CD40 and CD154 can be regarded as important target molecules in allograft rejection. The clinical development of the corresponding biological (humanized monoclonal anti-CD154) antibodies, however was previously thwarted by serious thromboembolic complications (Kawai et al., 2000; Koyama et al., 2004), which are suspected to have been caused by an interference with the stabilizing effect of soluble CD154 on freshly formed thrombi (Andre et al., 2002). In fact, the main source of soluble CD154 are aggregating platelets from which the membrane-bound CD154 is shed upon activation (Kaya et al., 2011; Pamukcu et al., 2011; Silvain et al., 2011; Yacoub et al., 2010). More recently, however, some progress has been made towards the development of monoclonal antibodies with less side effects (Hussein et al., 2010).

CD40 is a cell surface receptor that belongs to the family of tumor necrosis factor receptors. It is mainly expressed on B-cells and antigen-presenting cells, but also on other non-immune cells such as vascular smooth muscle cells, fibroblasts and endothelial cells (van Kooten & Banchereau, 2000; Schonbeck & Libby, 2001). The corresponding ligand, CD154, is a member of the TNF family and located on activated T-cells, dendritic cells, mast cells, eosinophils, activated platelets and endothelial cells (Cho et al., 2000). CD40 stimulation in endothelial cells elicits a marked increase in expression of adhesion molecules and chemokines, which in turn facilitate the extravasation of leukocytes and their accumulation in the inflamed tissue (Hollenbaugh et al., 1995; Yellin et al., 1995). In addition, endothelial cells, as APCs, produce interleukin-12 (IL-12) in response to CD40 stimulation, which may play a crucial role in strengthening the T-cell response during graft rejection (Ode-Hakim et al., 1996; D'Elios et al., 1997). This IL-12 production is strongly enhanced in the presence of IFN-γ.

7. STAT-1 decoy ODN treatment to ameliorate cardiac allograft survival

Since targeting CD154 therapeutically appears to be wrought with difficulties, CD40 may be the more suitable drug target. However, low-molecular-weight CD40 antagonists are not yet available and CD40 antibodies, although prolonging graft survival in earlier studies, may cause anti-antibody formation and anaphylaxis (Imai et al., 2007). Therefore, an alternative approach was sought addressing transcription of the CD40 gene in endothelial cells, and this was achieved by employing decoy ODNs directed against the transcription factor STAT-1.

To investigate this novel therapeutic concept in terms of acute and chronic graft rejection, STAT-1 decoy ODNs were applied in established models of allogeneic cardiac transplantation in rats and mice with or without immunosuppression and in both acute and chronic settings (Holschermann et al., 2006; Stadlbauer et al., 2008; Stojanovic et al., 2009). The exclusive uptake of the decoy ODNs by the donor coronary endothelium could be confirmed by administration of fluorescent dye-labelled nucleic acids. Given the pleiotropic influence of

CD154/CD40 expression and of IFN-γ on pro-inflammatory gene expression and the putative beneficial effect of STAT-1 decoy ODNs, the up-regulation of important chemokines and adhesion molecules was examined in cardiac allografts following periprocedural STAT-1 decoy ODN administration. To this end the expression of, e.g. CD40, VCAM-1, E-selectin, MCP-1, ICAM-1 and RANTES (Holschermann et al., 2006; Stojanovic et al., 2009) was analyzed. Furthermore, histological parameters of rejection and the profile of infiltrating inflammatory cells were monitored (Holschermann et al., 2006; Stadlbauer et al., 2008; Stojanovic et al., 2009).

As verified by real time PCR analysis, a single periprocedural application of STAT-1 decoy ODNs to the coronary arteries of allogeneic donor heart transplants resulted in a marked down-regulation of CD40, VCAM-1, E-selectin, MCP-1, ICAM-1 and RANTES expression in allografts but not in isografts 24 hours post transplantation when compared to allograft and isograft control hearts (Stojanovic et al., 2009). The corresponding mutant control ODNs showed no such effect on expression of these marker genes (Holschermann et al., 2006; Stojanovic et al., 2009).

In fact, expression of these gene products was even lower than in control syngeneic transplants. Moreover, in syngenic transplants, irrespective of the chosen treatment regimen, no change in the expression of CD40, ICAM-1 or MCP-1 was noted, but an increase in E-selectin and VCAM-1 expression occurred which probably is the consequence of a moderate surgical and ischemia/reperfusion trauma (Stojanovic et al., 2009). The expression of the aforementioned pro-inflammatory gene products in the allograft is IFN-γ-dependent and controlled by subsequent activation of the transcription factor STAT-1 (De Caterina et al., 2001; Burysek et al., 2002; Wagner et al., 2002). In addition, some of these pro-inflammatory gene products, e.g. MCP-1, regulate the expression of other pro-inflammatory genes (Saiura et al., 2004), so that a blockade of IFN-γ-induced MCP-1 expression through STAT-1 decoy ODN treatment probably could affect a much larger spectrum of pro-inflammatory gene products.

Besides MCP-1, which was still up-regulated 9 days after transplantation in the allografts compared with syngeneic transplanted hearts, there were no long-term changes in gene expression found in the donor hearts, so that the possible inhibitory effect of the STAT-1 decoy ODN treatment was no longer detectable at this time (Stojanovic et al., 2009).

When analyzing the profile of infiltrating cells, it was readily apparent that the number of infiltrating monocytes/macro-phages and T-cells was significantly reduced 6 days and 9 days post transplantation as compared to the allogeneic controls (Holschermann et al., 2006; Stojanovic et al., 2009). In line with these findings, the vascular and interstitial rejection scores were significantly reduced in STAT-1 decoy ODN-treated allografts 9 days post transplantation when compared to control allografts (Stojanovic et al., 2009), and accordingly a significantly prolonged graft survival was noted after single STAT-1 decoy ODN treatment in an allogeneic rat model (Holschermann et al., 2006).

This approach of specific interference with transcriptional regulation of gene expression by using decoy ODNs also holds true when targeting other key molecules involved in CD40 expression. Thus decoy ODNs directed against the transcription factor AP-1 also inhibited endothelial ICAM-1 and VCAM-1 expression and reduced the number of leukocytes, namely T-cells, infiltrating the graft blood vessels, and prolonged survival in acute rejection of cardiac allografts (Holschermann et al., 2006).

Analyzing the course of chronic rejection after single application of either a STAT-1 or AP-1 decoy ODN in a rat cardiac transplantation model with immunosuppression revealed that after 100 days allografts treated with either decoy ODN showed a significantly lesser degree of disease and number of occluded vessels, pointing towards a profound inhibition of cardiac allograft vasculopathy (CAV) (Stadlbauer et al., 2008). As putative mechanism of action, it was proposed that the AP-1 decoy ODN primarily attenuated basal endothelial CD40 expression while the STAT-1 decoy ODN suppressed tumour necrosis factor-α/IFN-γ-stimulated expression of CD40 in the rat native endothelial cells (Stadlbauer et al., 2008).

In the setting of inflammatory disease in humans another or perhaps alternative mechanism of CD40 expression in endothelial cells may also be active. In human cultured endothelial cells, combined treatment with IFN-γ and TNF-α induces an IRF-1–dependent *de novo* expression of CD40. Although this effect is indirectly mediated by STAT-1 through induction of IRF-1 synthesis, STAT-1 directly induces CD40 expression in these cells when exposed to IFN-γ alone. Thus, it is the cytokine composition under the given pro-inflammatory conditions that determines which transcription factor is primarily responsible for the increase in endothelial CD40 expression (Wagner et al., 2002).

8. Conclusion

The primary injury inflicted on the graft before implantation actually takes place currently does not receive sufficient attention. The mechanisms of innate immunity, which are significantly contributing to primary graft damage, are also not well understood, but at least regained scientific interest.

Herein an attempt was made to highlight some consequences of the inadvertently exaggerated activation of the innate immune response in cardiac transplant rejection with special emphasis on the role of the donor endothelium and the underlying pro-inflammatory mechanisms. By blocking the expression of pro-inflammatory gene products in these cells beneficial effects on the perfusion of the graft and its histological appearance can be achieved. The tested animal experimental models did not comprise a conventional immunosuppressive treatment regimen with regard to acute rejection and despite the fully allogeneic transplantation setting. There is the distinct possibility therefore that combining conventional immunosuppressive therapy with the presented novel decoy ODN drug approach results in an adequate immunosuppression with much less toxicity and a significantly better outcome with respect to long-term transplant function and survival. We believe that the underlying mechanism of action of these nucleic acid-based drugs can spur a promising field of research with midterm clinical implementation as a procurable perspective.

9. Acknowledgments

The authors are indebted to Dr. Gerd König for providing the figures and for critically reading of the manuscript. They are supported by the German Research Foundation (DFG), the Federal Ministry of Education and Research (BMBF), the European Commission and the German Cardiac Society (DGK).

10. References

Andre, P., K. S. Prasad, et al. (2002). "CD40L stabilizes arterial thrombi by a beta3 integrin--dependent mechanism." *Nat Med* 8(3): 247-52.

Azuma, H., L. C. Paul, et al. (1996). "Insights into acute and chronic rejection." *Transplant Proc* 28(4): 2081-4.

Bach, E. A., M. Aguet, et al. (1997). "The IFN gamma receptor: a paradigm for cytokine receptor signaling." *Annu Rev Immunol* 15: 563-91.

Boehm, U., T. Klamp, et al. (1997). "Cellular responses to interferon-gamma." *Annu Rev Immunol* 15: 749-95.

Burysek, L., T. Syrovets, et al. (2002). "The serine protease plasmin triggers expression of MCP-1 and CD40 in human primary monocytes via activation of p38 MAPK and janus kinase (JAK)/STAT signaling pathways." *J Biol Chem* 277(36): 33509-17.

Cho, C. S., M. M. Hamawy, et al. (2000). "CD40:CD154 interactions and allograft rejection." *Current Opinion in Organ Transplantation* 5: 10–15.

Christopher, K., T. F. Mueller, et al. (2002). "Analysis of the innate and adaptive phases of allograft rejection by cluster analysis of transcriptional profiles." *J Immunol* 169(1): 522-30.

D'Elios, M. M., R. Josien, et al. (1997). "Predominant Th1 cell infiltration in acute rejection episodes of human kidney grafts." *Kidney Int* 51(6): 1876-84.

Darnell, J. E., Jr. (1997). "STATs and gene regulation." *Science* 277(5332): 1630-5.

De Caterina, R., T. Bourcier, et al. (2001). "Induction of endothelial-leukocyte interaction by interferon-gamma requires coactivation of nuclear factor-kappaB." *Arterioscler Thromb Vasc Biol* 21(2): 227-32.

Dykstra, M., A. Cherukuri, et al. (2003). "Location is everything: lipid rafts and immune cell signaling." *Annu Rev Immunol* 21: 457-81.

Game, D. S. and R. I. Lechler (2002). "Pathways of allorecognition: implications for transplantation tolerance." *Transpl Immunol* 10(2-3): 101-8.

Ganster, R. W., B. S. Taylor, et al. (2001). "Complex regulation of human inducible nitric oxide synthase gene transcription by Stat 1 and NF-kappa B." *Proc Natl Acad Sci U S A* 98(15): 8638-43.

Gudmundsdottir, H. and L. A. Turka (1999). "T cell costimulatory blockade: new therapies for transplant rejection." *J Am Soc Nephrol* 10(6): 1356-65.

Hancock, W. W. (1999). "Current trends in transplant immunology." *Curr Opin Nephrol Hypertens* 8(3): 317-24.

He, H., J. R. Stone, et al. (2002). "Analysis of robust innate immune response after transplantation in the absence of adaptive immunity." *Transplantation* 73(6): 853-61.

He, H., J. R. Stone, et al. (2003). "Analysis of differential immune responses induced by innate and adaptive immunity following transplantation." *Immunology* 109(2): 185-96.

Hemmi, H. and S. Akira (2005). "TLR signalling and the function of dendritic cells." *Chem Immunol Allergy* 86: 120-35.

Hollenbaugh, D., N. Mischel-Petty, et al. (1995). "Expression of functional CD40 by vascular endothelial cells." *J Exp Med* 182(1): 33-40.

Hölschermann, H., T. H. Stadlbauer, et al. (2006). "STAT-1 and AP-1 decoy oligonucleotide therapy delays acute rejection and prolongs cardiac allograft survival." *Cardiovasc Res* 71(3): 527-36.

http://www.americanheart.org/presenter.jhtml?identifier=4588.
Hussein, M., J. R. Berenson, et al. (2010). "A phase I multidose study of dacetuzumab (SGN-40; humanized anti-CD40 monoclonal antibody) in patients with multiple myeloma." *Haematologica* 95(5): 845-8.
Ihle, J. N. (1996). "STATs: signal transducers and activators of transcription." *Cell* 84(3): 331-4.
Imai, A., T. Suzuki, et al. (2007). "A novel fully human anti-CD40 monoclonal antibody, 4D11, for kidney transplantation in cynomolgus monkeys." *Transplantation* 84(8): 1020-8.
Ishitani, T., G. Takaesu, et al. (2003). "Role of the TAB2-related protein TAB3 in IL-1 and TNF signaling." *Embo J* 22(23): 6277-88.
Ivashkiv, L. B. (1995). "Cytokines and STATs: how can signals achieve specificity?" *Immunity* 3(1): 1-4.
Janeway, C. A., Jr. and R. Medzhitov (2002). "Innate immune recognition." *Annu Rev Immunol* 20: 197-216.
Karonitsch, T., E. Feierl, et al. (2009). "Activation of the interferon-gamma signaling pathway in systemic lupus erythematosus peripheral blood mononuclear cells." *Arthritis Rheum* 60(5): 1463-71.
Kawai, T., D. Andrews, et al. (2000). "Thromboembolic complications after treatment with monoclonal antibody against CD40 ligand." *Nat Med* 6(2): 114.
Kaya, Z., K. Ozdemir, et al. (2011). "Soluble CD40 ligand levels in acute pulmonary embolism: a prospective, randomized, controlled study." *Heart Vessels* (DOI 10.1007/s00380-011-0142-4).
Khabar, K. S., L. Al-Haj, et al. (2004). "Expressed gene clusters associated with cellular sensitivity and resistance towards anti-viral and anti-proliferative actions of interferon." *J Mol Biol* 342(3): 833-46.
Khabar, K. S. and H. A. Young (2007). "Post-transcriptional control of the interferon system." *Biochimie* 89(6-7): 761-9.
Kirk, A. D., L. C. Burkly, et al. (1999). "Treatment with humanized monoclonal antibody against CD154 prevents acute renal allograft rejection in nonhuman primates." *Nat Med* 5(6): 686-93.
Kishida, S., H. Sanjo, et al. (2005). "TAK1-binding protein 2 facilitates ubiquitination of TRAF6 and assembly of TRAF6 with IKK in the IL-1 signaling pathway." *Genes Cells* 10(5): 447-54.
Koyama, I., T. Kawai, et al. (2004). "Thrombophilia associated with anti-CD154 monoclonal antibody treatment and its prophylaxis in nonhuman primates." *Transplantation* 77(3): 460-2.
Land, W. G. (2003). "Allograft injury mediated by reactive oxygen species: from conserved proteins of Drosophila to acute and chronic rejection of human transplants. Part III: Interaction of (oxidative) stress-induced heat shock proteins with Toll-like receptor-bearing cells of innate immunity and its consequences for the development of acute and chronic allograft rejection." *Transplantation Rev* 17: 67-86.
Land, W. G. (2005). "The role of postischemic reperfusion injury and other nonantigen-dependent inflammatory pathways in transplantation." *Transplantation* 79(5): 505-14.

Land, W. G. (2007). "Innate immunity-mediated allograft rejection and strategies to prevent it." *Transplant Proc* 39(3): 667-72.
Land, W. G. (2007). "Innate immunity-mediated allograft rejection and strategies to prevent it." *Transplant Proc* 39(3): 667-72.
LaRosa, D. F., A. H. Rahman, et al. (2007). "The innate immune system in allograft rejection and tolerance." *J Immunol* 178(12): 7503-9.

Larsen, C. P., P. J. Morris, et al. (1990). "Migration of dendritic leukocytes from cardiac allografts into host spleens. A novel pathway for initiation of rejection." *J Exp Med* 171(1): 307-14.

Larsen, C. P. and T. C. Pearson (1997). "The CD40 pathway in allograft rejection, acceptance, and tolerance." *Curr Opin Immunol* 9(5): 641-7.

Le Moine, A., M. Goldman, et al. (2002). "Multiple pathways to allograft rejection." *Transplantation* 73(9): 1373-81.

Liu, X., L. Ye, et al. (2008). "Activation of the JAK/STAT-1 signaling pathway by IFN-gamma can down-regulate functional expression of the MHC class I-related neonatal Fc receptor for IgG." *J Immunol* 181(1): 449-63.

Manes, S., G. del Real, et al. (2003). "Pathogens: raft hijackers." *Nat Rev Immunol* 3(7): 557-68.

Methe, H., S. Hess, et al. (2007). "Endothelial cell-matrix interactions determine maturation of dendritic cells." *Eur J Immunol* 37(7): 1773-84.

Mollen, K. P., R. J. Anand, et al. (2006). "Emerging paradigm: toll-like receptor 4-sentinel for the detection of tissue damage." *Shock* 26(5): 430-7.

Morishita, R., G. H. Gibbons, et al. (1995). "A gene therapy strategy using a transcription factor decoy of the E2F binding site inhibits smooth muscle proliferation in vivo." *Proc Natl Acad Sci U S A* 92(13): 5855-9.

Naik, S. M., N. Shibagaki, et al. (1997). "Interferon gamma-dependent induction of human intercellular adhesion molecule-1 gene expression involves activation of a distinct STAT protein complex." *J Biol Chem* 272(2): 1283-90.

Nakahira, K., H. P. Kim, et al. (2006). "Carbon monoxide differentially inhibits TLR signaling pathways by regulating ROS-induced trafficking of TLRs to lipid rafts." *J Exp Med* 203(10): 2377-89.

Ode-Hakim, S., W. D. Docke, et al. (1996). "Delayed-type hypersensitivity-like mechanisms dominate late acute rejection episodes in renal allograft recipients." *Transplantation* 61(8): 1233-40.

Pamukcu, B., G. Y. Lip. Et al., (2011). "The CD40-CD40L system in cardiovascular disease." *Ann Med* 43(5): 331-40.

Pestka, S. (1997). "The interferon receptors." *Semin Oncol* 24(3 Suppl 9): S9-18-S9-40.

Quarcoo, D., S. Weixler, et al. (2004). "Inhibition of signal transducer and activator of transcription 1 attenuates allergen-induced airway inflammation and hyperreactivity." *J Allergy Clin Immunol* 114(2): 288-95.

Reul, R. M., J. C. Fang, et al. (1997). "CD40 and CD40 ligand (CD154) are coexpressed on microvessels in vivo in human cardiac allograft rejection." *Transplantation* 64(12): 1765-74.

Rocha, P. N., T. J. Plumb, et al. (2003). "Effector mechanisms in transplant rejection." *Immunol Rev* 196: 51-64.

Rose, M. L. (1997). "Role of endothelial cells in allograft rejection." *Vasc Med* 2(2): 105-14.

Rose, M. L. (1998). "Endothelial cells as antigen-presenting cells: role in human transplant rejection." *Cell Mol Life Sci* 54(9): 965-78.

Russo, M. J., A. Iribarne, et al. (2010) "Factors associated with primary graft failure after heart transplantation." *Transplantation* 90(4): 444-50.

Saiura, A., M. Sata, et al. (2004). "Antimonocyte chemoattractant protein-1 gene therapy attenuates graft vasculopathy." *Arterioscler Thromb Vasc Biol* 24(10): 1886-90.

Sato, S., H. Sanjo, et al. (2005). "Essential function for the kinase TAK1 in innate and adaptive immune responses." *Nat Immunol* 6(11): 1087-95.

Schönbeck, U. and P. Libby (2001). "The CD40/CD154 receptor/ligand dyad." *Cell Mol Life Sci* 58(1): 4-43.

Shim, J. H., C. Xiao, et al. (2005). "TAK1, but not TAB1 or TAB2, plays an essential role in multiple signaling pathways in vivo." *Genes Dev* 19(22): 2668-81.

Silvain, J., J. P. Collet, et al. (2011). "Composition of coronary thrombus in acute myocardial infarction." *J Am Coll Cardiol* 57(12): 1359-67.

Stadlbauer, T. H., A. H. Wagner, et al. (2008). "AP-1 and STAT-1 decoy oligodeoxynucleotides attenuate transplant vasculopathy in rat cardiac allografts." *Cardiovasc Res* 79(4): 698-705.

Stojanovic, T., A. H. Wagner, et al. (2009). "STAT-1 decoy oligodeoxynucleotide inhibition of acute rejection in mouse heart transplants." *Basic Res Cardiol* 104(6): 719-29.

Takeda, K. and S. Akira (2005). "Toll-like receptors in innate immunity." *Int Immunol* 17(1): 1-14.

The International Society of Heart and Lung Transplantation guidelines for the care of heart transplant recipients Task Force 2:Immunosuppression and Rejection (Nov.8, www.ishlt.org/ContentDocuments/ISHLT_GL_TaskForce2_110810.pdf. from The International Society of Heart and Lung Transplantation guidelines for the care of heart transplant recipients Task Force 2:Immunosuppression and Rejection (Nov.8,2010), www.ishlt.org/ContentDocuments/ISHLT_GL_TaskForce2_110810.pdf.

van Kooten, C. and J. Banchereau (2000). "CD40-CD40 ligand." *J Leukoc Biol* 67(1): 2-17.

Wagner, A. H., M. Gebauer, et al. (2002). "Cytokine-inducible CD40 expression in human endothelial cells is mediated by interferon regulatory factor-1." *Blood* 99(2): 520-5.

Yacoub, D., A. Hachem, et al. (2010). "Enhanced levels of soluble CD40 ligand exacerbate platelet aggregation and thrombus formation through a CD40-dependent tumor necrosis factor receptor-associated factor-2/Rac1/p38 mitogen-activated protein kinase signaling pathway." *Arterioscler Thromb Vasc Biol* 30(12): 2424-33.

Yellin, M. J., J. Brett, et al. (1995). "Functional interactions of T cells with endothelial cells: the role of CD40L-CD40-mediated signals." *J Exp Med* 182(6): 1857-64.